D1579532

FIT TO FIGHT

PETER CONSTERDINE

PROTECTION PUBLICATIONS

FIT TO FIGHT

Copyright © Peter Consterdine 1996
Reprinted 2008

All rights reserved.

No part of this book may be reproduced by any means, nor transmitted, nor translated into a machine language without the written permission of the publisher.

Protection Publications,
4 Newmarket Mews,
Castle Gate,
Stanley,
Wakefield WF3 4AL.

A CIP catalogue record for this book is available from the British Library.

Printed and bound in Great Britain by J H Haynes & Co Ltd, Sparkford, Yeovil, Somerset BA22 7JJ
Typesetting: Protection Publications, Leeds.
Photographic Scanning & Output: Protection Publications, Leeds.
Cover Design & Origination: Art Style, Doncaster.

ISBN 0-9537638-0-3

Please note: The author and the publishers cannot accept any responsibility for any proceedings or prosecutions brought or instituted against any person or body as a result of the use or misuse of any techniques described in this book or any loss, injury or damage caused thereby.

Important Note
If you have or believe you have a medical condition, the exercises outlined in this book should not be attempted without first consulting your doctor. Some of the exercises in this book require a high level of fitness and suppleness and should not be attempted by someone lacking such fitness.

ACKNOWLEDGEMENTS

I would like to thank all those who have contributed their time to the photos in this book, with special thanks to:-

Tony and Bob Sykes at Colne Valley Black Belt Academy
Ged Moran and his people at Salford Shotokan
Pierre Mahon and his people at Wakefield Thai Boxing Camp
Aidan and Howard Greensmith at Sporting Bodies, Wakefield
Alan Bardsley - XED, Manchester
and last but not least my good friend and partner Geoff Thompson

Also my thanks to those people, some of whom I've acknowledged within the book, with whom I've trained and trained hard over many years.

"WHAT DOESN'T KILL US, MAKES US STRONG"

(Frederich Nietsche)

FIT TO FIGHT

CONTENTS Page

PREFACE

I started training in traditional Karate when I was 15, which for those people who don't know me, is a 'tad' over 10 years ago (for those that do, it's more like 35 years ago). Some 3-4 years later I was firmly entrenched on the Gt. Britain and England Karate squad. I had firmly resisted traditional school sports throughout my academic life, but threw myself into the rigours of Karate and, with the best of them, marched up and down throwing kicks, punches and blocks with mind numbing intensity. Other training was fairly non-existent and it wasn't until, in my late teens, that the feeling that I needed more, came into being. This coincided with my starting work 'on the doors' in Manchester, where I stayed at one club for some six years.

This particular club grew over the years to become a cavernous affair, being split over two floors and having a capacity in excess of a thousand people. From the door to the furthest room was nearly halfway across Manchester, albeit underground. The system used to summon us from the door to a trouble spot, was the same as used in countless nightclubs, that is a loud bell and a flashing light, indicating which room the trouble was in and whether one was being summoned by the DJ in that room or by someone at the bar who had seen the trouble flair.

For those of you who have never had the dubious pleasure of 'working the doors', it acquaints closely, I would think, with the life of a Fireman - long periods of boring inactivity, punctuated by short bursts of panic, stress and sometimes terror. The starting point is the same - the sound of the bell.

The sound of the bell going off was not simply a detached signal that indicated you were required somewhere at your leisure. It was 'Pavlovian' - and although it didn't produce a salivating effect, as the bell did with Pavlov's dogs, the reaction we experienced, instantaneously triggered off that huge 'dump' of adrenalin, instant nerves, rapidly increased heartrate, tension and trepidation. All the emotions and clinical responses became mixed and were then exacerbated by exertion.

With a single glance at the bell board, everyone 'set off'. Two or more doormen took the first few steps in one bound and then set off what can only be described as a human obstacle race, bouncing off corridor walls, missing and not missing people in the way, taking stairs four or more at a time and negotiating past hundreds of people. With a heart rate touching two hundred, one would eventually reach the scene of the action.

Often whatever had happened had been over for some time, which was inevitable given the time we took to get there, or we would have to fight. With your legs 'gone solid' and shaking with exertion, an inability to talk due to gasping for breath and a lead ball in your stomach the size of some-

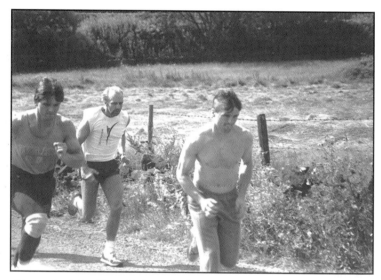

From the left - Tony Sykes, Author, and Bob Sykes, hillsprinting, Huddersfield - early '90s. Sprinting and hill work have been my core training for 25 years plus.

thing that sank the Armada, the chances of being effective were greatly diminished. It was on these occasions that I came to realise that if I ever had to seriously run from or to a fight, that I was ill-prepared and that when it came to the hands and legs bit, that I probably wouldn't have it. What I realised above everything was that the majority of my training was not done under 'STRESS' conditions, which is the real world. To be fair, I had thought for some time that my internal reserves lacked a certain depth, but what struck me the most was how much more reluctant I was to engage in a fight when I felt distressed, as I knew how taxing it would become and I knew that how I would feel was weakening my resolve. I always wanted to feel 'comfortable' and in control of combat situations. I didn't want to engage in combat, feeling as if I'd just come from a 15-round fight. I wasn't physically prepared sufficiently to deal with the reality of the situation.

From early on working the door, I had quickly come to the realisation that in order to survive, it was necessary to develop a strategy of Pre-emptiveness, when one knew that a fight was probably inevitable, but in the early days I didn't always get it right and often found myself in a brawl. When this happens, all the 'anti-success' agents come to the fore - fear, adrenalin, lactic acid, dead legs, hollow stomach and a waining mental resolve.

I knew that I needed to train outside the confines of Karate and it took many years of self-discipline, pursuing a variety of training routes and methods, both with others and by myself, to establish a wide range of drills and skills to achieve what I needed. I now know that in the event of **flight or fight** that I may end up wth those same debilitating feelings, but I also know that I can fight through. I've been there plenty of times and know how to plumb the depths. From better understanding the clinical responses, I can also put my 'emotions' and feelings into convenient boxes. I no longer confuse the feeling of fear and adrenalin for example. I also know that my opponent is feeling equally as bad and that we are usually only seconds away from one of us quitting, but I know without reservation that in the street it won't be me.

I know that when I'm on a hill with someone on my back that I'll make it those last few feet to the top, however bad I'm feeling. Some days you won't make it through a training session for whatever reason, but what you also know is that on those days when you're having a bad one, that if you don't succeed today, you'll be back tomorrow and make up for it.

You should be intimidated by your training sessions, not every one, but at least two or three out of four to five in a week. If you're not intimidated by these special sessions then they're not hard enough.

You should literally find it hard to sleep the night before. These sessions may be on the hills, or in the Dojo or Gym, but wherever, they should be so hard that only very few people will consistantly train with you.

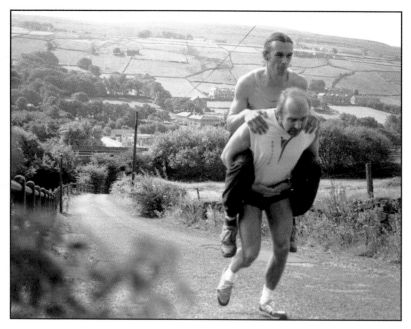

A long hill carry. Very few people will consistantly turn out to train at this level of intensity. Hill carries are like training - "you're either going up and its hard or you're going down - there's no middle ground".

Over the years I've had excellent training partners and I've always managed to associate myself with people who were never satisfied with coasting along or making do, but people who would always make a session hard if they were in charge, or go along with my regime if it was me who took the lead. The one thing you must have in a partner is consistency - someone who will be ready on time, come hell or bad weather and who is ready to train, not just take part. Everyone can't feel world beating all the time, but however you feel, you must NEVER allow any negativity you feel to influence others. Be positive and aggressive and leave your ego at home.

I've seen senior martial artists whose ego can't take the severity of hard physical training. Whatever grade you are, (which is bollocks anyway) if you can't hack a hard 'cross training' regime you need to look at yourself. You practise a combat system and it's a disgrace to see supposed senior martial artists look like they've spread like a 'bag of wet cement'.

Also over the years I've been happy to align myself with people of whatever grade, in whatever system, who I know will push me to the limits. I don't like it because I'm intimidated by failure or the prospect and I'm intimidated by not doing well in front of others, but generally I'll never let myself down. I know I've got enough depth of self and control of my ego to come back for more if it was hard and intimidating the first time.

In the early 80's I was training with Lance Lewis and Brian Seabright, both of whom were British Full Contact Champions, boxers and natural martial artists. Amongst other things they were into two minute rounds of kicking on the body shields, which up to that time I had simply been using for power kicking. I remember the first session where my thighs seized up and I wobbled down four flights of stairs to leave the building. However over the following months and subsequent years I was able to not only complete the drills, but ensure that the rounds on the shields were full power ones as well.

I've never been 'hamstrung' by being a natural. By that I mean I realised very early on that I was not naturally fit, naturally strong nor naturally talented from a sporting aspect. I realised that only repetition and hard work would ever allow me to be good and, in some areas, marginally above good, but I also realised more than anything that to work hard would be a constant mental battle with myself and my own worst instincts.

Training is like pushing a stalled car uphill. You're either going up or your rolling down, there's no half way. Either your working hard and pushing yourself all the time or you're not and your making excuses and your fitness is lost. The middle ground which I say doesn't exist does - it exists in peoples minds!, who deceive themselves that they are still pushing it They say to you, upon enquiry, that they are *"holding their own",* or they're into a period of 'maintenance' - bollocks- they're rolling backwards and need to be honest enough to see it. I know when it happens to me and I've learned to let my conscience have free reign.

So - this book is NOT written by someone to whom training comes easy and who was born with natural talent. This book is written, however, by someone who has worked harder than most, for longer than many and who is prepared to put himself in intimidating training situations.

> ## *"MAINTAIN AN ARMY FOR A THOUSAND YEARS, IF ONLY TO FIGHT FOR ONE DAY"*
>
> ### *(Ancient Chinese Proverb)*

INTRODUCTION

This book is not primarily about fitness, rather it is about winning fights. It is about developing a winning attitude and about developing an indomitable spirit. The fights you may be keen to win could be in a ring, on a Dojo mat or, more critically, in the street. But, wherever they take place and why you are there are all secondary to winning.

To achieve success in a fight is the sum total of many physical aspects and attributes, both technique and training related, but the deciding factor in terms of a successful outcome is solely related to one factor only - 'mental attitude'. This can often be the missing link for many people who find themselves confronted in the street with an intimidating, aggressive, threatening and often frightening confrontation. Don't believe that being a high grade in martial arts lessens any of these emotions and often they are heightened due to a fear of failure should things go wrong when years of training seem to go down the drain. One pound for every martial artist whose been taken out in the street or knocked out on the door would swell a bank account to very enviable proportions.

For many martial artists, they never experience the stark reality of real combat until it is too late. This book is not about developing a complete approach to surviving street confrontations (see the authors book **'Streetwise'**), it is about one piece of the jigsaw. It is about the mental edge and attitude that can be bred through the physical exertions of hard training and conditioning. Hard, demanding physical training is not about developing strength, speed or suppleness, although these elements and a good cardio-vascular capacity are part of what one should aim for. More importantly, it is about the effect it has on a persons mental attitude and the consequent mental control that we exercise over ourselves.

The physical aspects and results of a training regime are transient. They will stay with you as long as they are maintained through exertion, but when that stops, years of training will not ensure that a persons fitness remains - it will leave your body in a matter of weeks as if a tap has been turned on. What can and does remain, however, is that mind set of winning, that attitude not to give up.

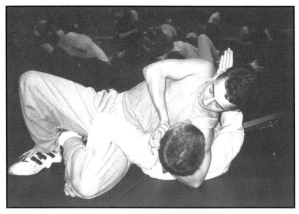

Grappling, in real life, will drain you in seconds if you're not fit.

Many years ago I enjoyed watching a business training video which centered around the business success of former American Football players who were ex-members of the **Green Bay Packers**. The Packers in the 60's, under the guidance of their then coach **Vince Lombardi**, enjoyed unrivalled success in the sport. Lombardi was successful because he understood what separated winners from losers. He knew it wasn't skill, physical prowess or strength and speed, rather he worked on his players mental strengths. He bred a desire and a will to win and recognised the transient nature of physical abilities, rather the permanent improvement in the 'positive' attitude that flowed from training.

He said; *"all the money, all the prizes, all the success linger in the memory for a few short years then are soon gone, but the will to win, the will to endure, that's what remains."*

How do we obtain that will to win though. For me it's attained by the constant re-inforcement of succeeding at hard training sessions. Training is not about easy workouts and perfecting technique and pleasant experiences and if your looking for a book that will pamper to the 'token trainer' in you then put this book back on the shelf. This book is not about how to build a programme of easy to do aerobic exercises - it is about plugging you into a taxing and hard to endure regime, which tests not only your physical capability, but, and this is the primary intent, your mental resources.

'**Fit to Fight**' is about **NOT GIVING UP** and this is the key to your success in winning fights. Fights are not lost because of bad technique. Once a fight starts and it's one you were unable to stop with pre-emptive action, (dialogue or a knockout), then the fight will not always be won by the fittest or strongest, but by the one with the stronger mind. By the same token, however, it's not sufficient to simply rely on a strong mind and neglect all the other aspects and, very much, this book will provide for you all the training drills you need to compliment a strong mind.

To give in on the street may be to suffer serious injury, or at worst, die. It's happening all the time and we read about such incidents daily. The scum who walk the streets these days revel in causing as much pain, suffering and injury to innocent people as they can. Violence has taken on a very gratuitious nature. Maiming or killing someone holds no fear for them and the 'pack' instincts getting stronger all the time. Unfortunately you cannot learn how not to give up during a fight by going and picking fights - it has to be derived elsewhere.

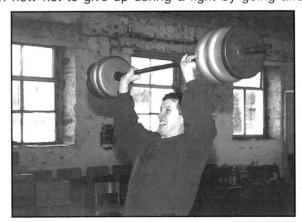

Not giving up in the gym, conditions us to not giving up in the street.

The feeling of hollow dread you experience prior to a fight and then the feeling of utter emptiness and dissipation of strength and energy during it, are in large part clinical in origin. These feelings are a combination of some psychological emotions such as fear and some physiological symptoms such as adrenalin and mild shock, but when they grip hold of you they will nullify whatever brilliant techniques you may have developed in the relative safety of the Dojo or the boxing or wrestling gym. One thing and one thing only will get you through those feelings and that's AGGRESSION. A controlled, fighting aggression must be developed and, unfortunately, it's not natural in most people. To develop it you must place yourself in 'Pressure' situations where only aggression and mental focus will see you through to successful conclusion in the endeavour.

When you feel confident to embark on some training drills in this book you will experience a very close approximation of the feeling of hollow inability to carry on, particularly with the heavy Anaerobic work, but you will know that in 'pushing through', your subconscious is being programmed to accept that however bad you feel you have that 'extra' mental surge in you. This, over a period, will build into an indomitable spirit, fed by controlled aggression.

Few of us are confident by nature. We become confident through the experience of success. Those people who suffer an attack in the street, usually unprovoked and often gratuitously violent, are never the same again. Their confidence in themselves and their abilities can be shattered forever. The techniques and concepts of Self Protection you will have to learn from elsewhere (see **Streetwise**), but the confidence and strength of purpose you can develop from severe training with induced stress, you will find in these pages.

Whatever you might be studying as a martial art or training in - weights, boxing etc, never lose sight of the fact that the physical returns on your effort are secondary to the development of 'Correct Attitude' that you are building. Don't ever believe that size and strength, however intimidating will win the day, nor, even, combat capability and there is a story which illustrates the fragility of personal belief. George Foreman, prior to one of his fights with Ali had the not inconsiderable advantage of having that great ring strategist Archie Moore employed by his camp to work with him. Moore later said that Foremans confidence - and remember this is one of the worlds greatest heavyweight boxers - was so precarious, that he used to let him win at 'ping pong' when they played so as not to shake his confidence in himself. Many people are beaten before the fight starts. They have no inate animal instinct to win and no 'trained' aggressive response to 'fight through'.

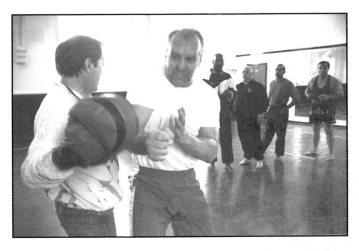

Build aggression on the pads - so you learn to turn it on and off as required.

This book is about training the spirit through the exertion of the body. You will be able to fill that hollow dread with the hot fire of aggression that you will gain from the training drills. To complete some of the drills we go through in this book is only possible as a result of being totally focused on one objective. This may be to complete a number of repetitions, reach the time determined for the exercise or reach the object you are sprinting to - possibly uphill. When your body has gone anaerobic, the lactic acid has set in and you're running on an empty tank, that tank must still be fuelled by something and that is your mind, which feeds in to your system sufficient aggression to get you to the end.

Some people who are reading this book may be martial artists, open minded enough to want to widen their knowledge or you may be someone who has no martial arts experience, but who feel they must do something to put them on a road to fitness, self-confidence and a path towards a combat system.

Do not get confused, however, this book is about fighting and I don't want anyone to loose sight of this. The drills and routines in this book have been developed from a variety of sources and have seen me through a traditional international Karate career, full contact fighting, years of doorwork and other combat and conflict situations. The routines are **'cross-applicable'.** They can be mixed and matched in most cases, although some of the more technical martial arts ones wont translate into the street, but the spirit from the application will. It's a book about fighting, because it's a book about mental domination, both of your opponent, but predominantly and certainly primarily oneself.

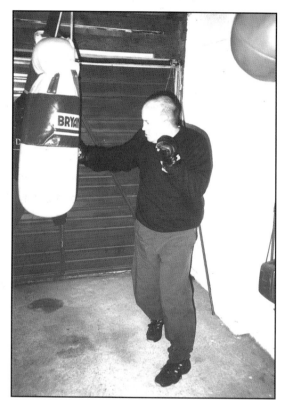

Geoff Thompson - my partner in the British Combat Asssociation and one of the hardest trainers I know.

YOU MUST KNOW YOURSELF TO HAVE ANY CHANCE OF WINNING OR THE ABILITY TO CHANGE!

CHAPTER I

MOTIVATION

As I mentioned in the Introduction, it's important that we know ourselves before we can make any changes or better understand why we act in certain ways, particularly if we have a desire to change how we act. To achieve any improvements in the way we act, that is our behaviour, we must first better understand the relationship between two separate, but connected matters - **Motivation and Emotions.** The two are inseparable in determining our behaviour. Broadly, Psychologists tell us that motivation is a general term for those feelings or forces that push and prod us to do something, whereas emotions refers to our subjective feelings or moods. Seldom will we ever be motivated to do anything however, without some underlying emotion such as fear or excitement or intense desire (not to fail in something for example), supplying the catalyst for the motivation to act in some way or other.

But how do we separate and understand the two. I realised many years ago that unless I better understood my motivations and what drove me, that I would never have any control over myself. This necessitated a great deal of study of basic psychology, with particular regard to behaviour and drive.

'Emotions give rise to motivations, give rise to behaviour', but remember, there are few consistencies. Performance one day, whilst excellent, may be mediocre the next - performance is not determined by either our learning, skills or abilities, but by our motivation and our self-belief at the time. If only skills were necessary for success, no golfer would ever have a bad day. Motivation is what makes our

behaviour and performance more than the sum parts of our physical abilities and learning sensations. This is not a book about psychology, but an understanding of the subject must be a part of our mental preparation.

We need to know what prompts us to action and probably more importantly, what stops us achieving the goal we want, be it in training or worse still, in the middle of a fight. Even when a person's life is one the line, they will simply run out of steam and give up, and in everyone at such a time, there can be found something in reserve if it can be dug out.

The study of psychology was dominated in the late 1800's and early 1900's by the Instinct Theory ie. that humans, just like certain species of animals, will behave in ways that are driven by millenia of instincts. There was a growing school of thought that proposed that humans were even more instinct driven, as they were also spurred on by a raft of psychological instincts such as jealousy, hate, fear, lust etc. From a list of 15 instincts proposed by Wm James in 1890, the list grew to over 15,000 by the 1920's.

Psychologists eventually realised the basic flaw in the Instinct Theory, in that instincts did not explain behaviour, rather they just gave a convenient way of labelling it and whilst genetic factors are recognised as having an influence, it is learning and experience which has a telling influence. A theory which is important to look at is **The Drive-Reduction Theory** - *"a drive is something unpleasant that motivates a being to engage in behaviour which reduces this unpleasant state of tension."*

Primary drives, ie the need for food and water helps us understand this concept, but are biological and don't arise from experience or learning. In contrast, 'secondary' or acquired drives do and may result in our need to work to reduce, say, fear or any unpleasant situation. The drive reduction theory is inadequate however, to deal with the huge range of human motivations, particularly those which are incentive based. The need for power or the need to achieve, fly in the face of the 'drive reduction theory', which states that the motivation will reduce as the goal is reduced. In reality, we know, once we achieve, we simply go on to achieve more and once we have power, we most definately strive to gain more. Incentive, not just drive, must also have a part to play in our motivations, and a psychologist called Abraham Maslow provided the most complex of theories of human motivation.

Basically he saw human motivation as a five block pyramid, the pemise being, that until the lower layer or motivation is satisfied, we do not and cannot be motivated by any of the factors higher up the scale. The bottom building block is made up of our physiological needs ie. food, water, air, which as basic biological needs, fits with the drive-reduction theory in that the absence of one or more motivates us to behaviour designed to remove the problem. And the absence of one of the biological factors would certainly prevent other motivations coming to the fore - as someone said *"it's hard to be motivated to achieve a better sprint time, when you're about to drown."* You want air, need air and will fight for air to the exclusion of all else.

The second block in the pyramid covers safety and security. Having satisfied the biological requirements, our motivations turn to such things as safety, security, warmth etc. Again, until these things are satisfied, our desire to want to secure a sense of love will be flawed. Moving up the pyramid, we come to esteem needs. This is our desire to want to achieve the highest level of competence and be the best - to achieve and be seen and recognised in that achievement. Self-actualisation is supposedly that state where we no longer need the approbation of others, but act in a selfless, altruistic way in our work for others.

Maslow's concept that we must fulfill our basic needs before we can pursue needs on a higher level make some sense, but as the years have gone by and it has proved difficult by empirical research to prove or not the theory, it has fallen into disuse, but for me it was a starting point to help understand what made me tick. Personally, although Maslow gave me a simple matrix for understanding certain drives, his theory seldom held good at all times, as there have often been times when, on his pyramid, the 'block below' has been in disrepair, yet I have been motivated to push ahead with some need to achieve! Often during those times of financial, business or personal stress, when a number of issues were substantially uncertain, I have worked or trained harder at those matters concerning self-esteem. This is one of the benefits of training and martial arts - that whatever else is going wrong, you always have these in which one can take comfort and security. Maybe self-esteem is the fly in the ointment of the theory, because when other things are going wrong, I train harder and in a way, am driven in this regard, not incentivised to do it.

This is one of the things we must understand, that often we will act in a certain way eg. hard training, but the source of the motivation is completely different. Somehow the emotional base from which the motivation has come has subtly altered. I believe we are either pushed towards or attracted to a goal, that is, we are either driven to it or we have an incentive which pulls us to the goal. It would be wrong to label one negative, say, in the case of the drive and one positive in the case of the incentive-based motivation, but whatever it is, we should know it so as to control ourselves better.

The motivation of Self-Esteem can probably be labelled positive or negative as we believe that the desire to want to do better, the want to win, the want to get that next grade is positive, whilst we perceive it as negative that some emotion drives us to NEED that self-esteem as a lifeboat in an otherwise turbulent sea of life. I personally recognise that both are very much present in my makeup and I no longer view either as positive or negative.

But by far the earliest and strongest emotion that stimulated motivation was fear. In my case it was a fear that I would lose fights from as early as I can remember - concern

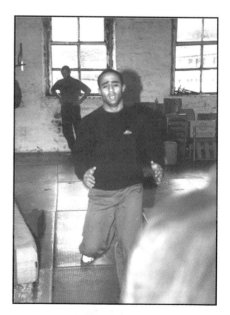

Self-esteem, means not quitting, however hard wind sprints get.

that other people were harder, more capable and more vicious than I was. As a motivating force, it has driven me, good or bad, to work harder than most to reduce that feeling and control the situation. As it has driven man himself to develop the ultimate in weaponry, whilst on an individual level, fear has driven me to train consistently at the highest level, so as to be better than the next man.

I summarised for myself some years ago how I saw my own motivation and it simplified into three areas:-

CONCERN
COMMITMENT
CONSCIENCE

Concern - that I cannot afford to let my training slip as I need to be better, faster, harder, stronger and more capable than the next man and for concern read fear.

Commitment - to myself, that to let up is letting my own self-image down and that the commitment to oneself is the only one that ultimately sustains you. Over the years I've relied on my commitment to others to get me to training sessions, as I know how difficult it is to train on ones own, but I've never lost sight of the fact that

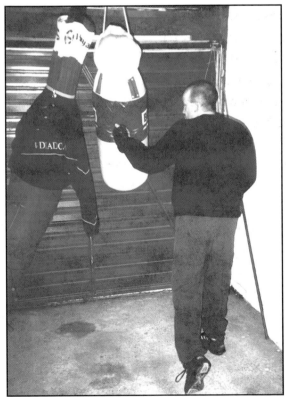

Concern - to be better than the next, means you must make the most of what you have - even if it means dressing up your punchbag!!

ultimately the time it will tell is when I've no-one to train with and the commitment is just with myself.

Conscience - in that, over the years, because of the habit forming mature of routine and the stress resulting from the importance I give to training, I am driven by conscience not to let up and miss sessions or tone down the degree of difficulty. If I don't get the number of hill sprints in one day because I feel so bad, I know how motivational my conscience is to drive me to achieve the next time.

So where do aspects like goals and enjoyment come into it? Quite simply they don't when it comes to the core training. With this training and the stress element, there is little enjoyment to be honest even on completion, it's a sense of relief as much as anything. I do take part in non stress, non-core training and do enjoy it eg. aerobics, step classes and things like 'boxercise' classes, but they are part of the 'aerobic' work and serve the mainly clinical need to keep fat levels down and cardiovascular capacity up.

Over the years I've been motivated, like many others in the martial arts world, to train for grades and trudged up that ladder until I realised that having ten dans wouldn't save me from being knocked out by someone who practised deceipt and had a good right hook. Chasing grades is at the bottom of the block of self esteem and it is striven for usually, so that a person can display it to others, more so than it ever is as a sign of achievement for oneself. Particularly these days, when there has crawled out of the woodwork, tenth dans and professors who couldn't hold their own against anyone but their own students who they set up - the whole system is devalued and false.

On the open page of hard training there is no hiding place, unlike the closed book of incompetence, and 'supposed' high grades who couldn't 'cut it' for an hour in a beginners 'step class'. Anyway, it's time to move on as I can feel the hairs on the back of my neck start to rise and the stomach starting to churn as I think about it. For me, my goals are now 'tactical' not 'strategic'. By this I mean that I have no long term goals in training, but rather I am motivated by achievement of set times, sets, repetitions and achieved levels of performance. I'm still driven rather than inspired.

Hope of Success versus Fear of Failure.

What determines whether we avoid a difficult task such as a hard physical training session or try our best to achieve it and what makes us set low goals which will never tax us - in this case say easy training sessions.

A number of researchers have theorised that our motive to achieve is the result of a complex battle between 'hope and success' and 'fear and failure'.

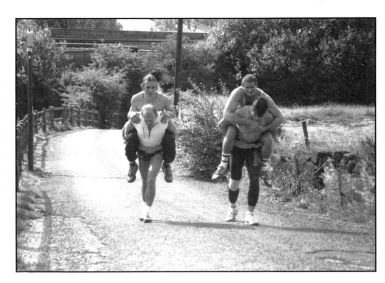

Hill Carries - for some training drills you obviously need partners to be able to do them, but more importantly, for this level of effort, you need mutual support.

The theory states that we may want to become involved in a task because we would like to succeed in it, but at the same time we may be repelled by a fear of failure - overall our net **'achievement motivation'** is seen as a result of the combination of these two interacting forces. Psychologists tell us that fear of failure influences task selection and the way of thinking and because two opposing processes are involved in 'achievement motivation', certain results will follow. The first of these is that those people who are motivated to avoid failure rather than strive for success will pursue goals, strangely, that are either very easy or, actually very difficult. The theory is that as the expectation is low for most people who take on difficult tasks, then those who fear failure will always hide within the fact that as the task was hard, there is no disgrace in losing.

The theory goes on to say that people will also avoid moderate tasks, as there is no hiding place if they do badly. People, however, motivated by hope or expectation or success are likely to set more realistic goals. Regrettably, I recognise a great deal of the first type in myself. I was always more concerned with the avoidance of losing than the inspiration of winning and that very irrational, but very strong motivation has been my motivation for a great deal of my work in the Combat Arts.

In the competition arena it limited me to being a good fighter, but never a great fighter. But this and other strong emotive sensations, make up my power source of motivation to train.

The same is going on with you, but unfortunately for many people, they never understand the source of their motivation, or lack of it and seldom, as a consequence, fulfill their potential. I submit though that if you don't know yourself well you will never sustain a commitment to hard training over many years. Driven or inspired, you should identify the emotive source and, if possible, harness that to give you focus. I am to all intents and purposes 'driven' and driven by those needs represented at the bottom end of Maslow's 'Pyramid of Human Needs' - to me security is as important as air, but what you must work hard at it to see where you fit.

Self-analysis requires, unfortunately, honesty and there are very few people who even if they are completely honest in every other area of their lives, can be honest about themselves. Barriers are erected to present to the outside world, with the image we want to portray, until eventually we begin to believe 'our own press releases'. Nowhere else, other than in the martial arts world, does this seem as prolific, which is probably why certain disfunctional people are drawn to it in the first place, but I know from my meeting them that there's more of the 'bullshitters' in this game than in any other I know.

"Energy follows thought" - Thoughts precede all our actions. Negative aspects of life eg a sudden threat, trigger an automatic psychological response which is the flight or fight syndrome.

The response produces **EMERGENCY CHEMICALS** - essentially these break down into other more toxic substances and are removed by the body creating huge physiological stresses

Group Dependent

Many people who I've seen over many years in the martial arts have functioned well within a group situation and achieved remarkable personal success. However when that group split or broke up the ability to sustain individual performance has been less than good.

The problem is that the motivation to train has been supplied by a mutually supportive, broadly, mutually singular goal driven arrangement, but on its dissolution, individuals find themselves unable to continue working at such a high level of demanding output. I've seen this happen with a number of individuals over the years. My view is we cannot afford to put ourselves in others' hands. We must be totally capable of sustaining a high output, within stressful situations, without a group goal and its mutual support. This is not to say that we never need training partners, rather that the role of the training partners in a group is strongly individual. Personally I don't want to be part of a 'team'. I don't want to win together or join a club, but what I do need are training partners, motivated by whatever emotions, to bring a synergy to group work that allows individuals to get more out of these sessions than they ever would on their own.

Encouragement, being pushed, being challenged, but more importantly, having yardsticks by which to measure our own performance is what group training is all about. Also, group training allows the inclusions of drills and exercises which more than double the potential range of exercises we can include in our training sessions. If you always train on your own, you're operating in a vacuum. You'll seldom know where you are on that psychological hill and as I said before, you need the yardstick of someone whose performance you know well, to know how good you are at any time.

Also, recognise and deal with laziness. Because I am a 'driven' trainer and not one inspired by higher ideals, I constantly fight mental battles as to whether I need to go and train, need to go out in the snow and rain, need to suffer on a grass slope, etc etc. The mental battles rage without my actual involvement, as they happen at a subconscious level without my consciously taking part, but its often touch and go who wins. Many years ago I found the answer in commitment. That is committing myself to someone else so that I had to be wherever at whatever time - ready to train. This is one of the benefits of training with others.

For many years at 9.30 every Sunday morning a good training friend of mine, Neil Rigby and I met to train for 2 hours. We had many people over the years who came and went, but nearly without fail, we were always there rain, shine, snow, shit - we'd train through it all. Neil was one of the most reliable partners I've ever had. Tony and Bob Sykes from Huddersfield are two other people to whom hard training is a way of life. My time training with them was some of the best I've had and stands out as one of the hardest all-round trainings which I could put alongside the years with Lance Lewis and Brian Seabright from Manchester.

Even 2 years on a remote corner of the west coast of Scotland found me with another excellent training partner, Tim Clifford, who would subject himself to every physical horror I could throw at him, but who like me, knew his own problems In maintaining solo effort. In Scotland I often had to dig deep to push myself on my own and many times didn't achieve the levels I would have liked, but whatever the result, I would go out for more. I ran more there (along the coastal roads) than I've ever done before and often into the teeth of a westerly wind that felt like I was pushing a bus. That wind would reduce a sprint to an old man's shuffle. I had every reason in Scotland not to train - I had no image to protect, no threat that big cities produce, yet I was driven to work and work hard, whether through commitment, attitude or years of conditioning, previous experience and to no small extent, conscience drove me on.

Beware, however, the problem of psychological dependence on exercise. Sports psychologists now recognise the problem and words such as 'obsessed', 'addicted' and 'compelled' are often applied. Chemical dependence, would seem a problem as the various chemicals released during training can have a very positive effect mentally. Balance is the key and recognising when training is getting out of hand to the extent that the other parts of your life suffer - family, work etc.

More is not always better! Even to the extent that serious injuries can occur and, particularly, the opposite of what one set out to achieve such as health and effectiveness at sport or combat begins to happen.

I want to mental edge that hard training gives me and I want the physical power, speed, technique and impact that I'll acquire, but more importantly I want the mental rewards that I can turn on aggression to push through and not give up.

> ## *"NO, WHEN THE FIGHT BEGINS WITHIN HIM-SELF A MAN'S WORTH SOMETHING"*
>
> ### *(Robert Browning)*

CHAPTER 2

FITNESS OVERVIEW

Fitness - what is it? Quite honestly it's anybody's guess. I'm continually astounded how the boundaries of human fitness and endurance are constantly pushed back. I watch the seeming, impossible efforts of the 'extreme' runners who tackle mountains in competitive races in a few hours. Anyone who has done any Fell Racing knows the degree of effort needed, but these people defy imagination.

Who would have thought, prior to 1978 - when U.S Marine Commander John Collins and some friends sat down with a beer in a bar in Honolulu, to argue who was the best endurance athletes- swimmers, cyclists, or runners - that people would actually now compete in 'Ironman' Triathlons, combining a 2.4 mile swim, 112 mile bike ride and a 26.2 mile run. Over 3 plus hours is now wiped off the times that Collins and his friends originally did it in, when they combined the then, individual events of the Waiki rough water swim, the Oahu bike ride and the Honolulu marathon. In the year 2000, Triathlon will become an Olympic event using the ITU 'short course' distances of 1500m swim, 40km bike ride and 10km run. We've come to accept it as a normal sporting event.

Aerobic capacity, strength, flexibility, speed, stamina, endurance, athleticism etc etc are all terms we hear used in regard to fitness. In some way each one has a part to play, however small, in every sport, but for most sports one aspect is emphasised over others. Some sports, by their very nature can be all things to all people as the intensity, by decreasing distance and increasing speed and power, create almost a different sport in the effect they have on the human body. The most stark example these days is the physical contrast between sprinters and marathon runners. Most top level sprinters wouldn't be out of place in a bodybuilding competition, yet they and their somewhat thinner marathon counterparts, practise the same discipline - running.

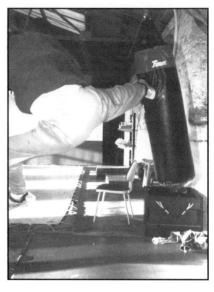

Bob Sykes - spinning back kick. This level of kicking demands every aspect of athleticism.

When our imperitives are formed by the need to be combative, the field narrows as to what degree, of which fitness aspects, we should concentrate on. I've covered this elsewhere, particularly with regard to running and if you had a choice of relevant sports to choose from you couldn't go far wrong with something like rowing. Strength, power, endurance - both muscular and cardio-vascular are all trained into Olympic rowers, combined with the most amazing mental focus and determination. Just what we need. Over the rest of this chapter I just want to look at some issues which I feel are important we should know about exercise in general. Some are purely for information and some are technique oriented.

The American College of Sports Medicine, has stated that, 'apparently', healthy individuals under age 45 can usually begin exercise programmes without the need for a physical examination. The proviso is, that the programme to be embarked upon begins and proceeds gradually and as long as the individual is alert to the development of unusual signs or symptoms of medical problems. Over 45, or if you are unsure, pay a visit to your GP - some use he'll be though!

Aerobic Capacity

Aerobic means simply 'with oxygen' and in aerobic exercise, oxygen is primarily involved in the metabolic process that produces energy. Optimum cardiovascular conditioning can be explained as *'training without straining'*. Anaerobic exercise, on the other hand, involves short bursts of intense effort and is fuelled by ATP (Adenosine Triphosphate) stored in the muscles (although only for a few seconds) and glycogen. Aerobic energy metabolism draws on both fat and glycogen. The longer you continue the exercise, the greater the body will have to rely on fat.

Broadly, we are training aerobically, if we exercise sufficiently to raise our heartbeat for 25 minutes or more. Such activities as running, rowing, cycling, tennis etc etc. can all be considered aerobic. A steady pace alone, will burn fat eventually, whilst an increased pace, for short periods will push the envelope of our aerobic capacity by working on our cardio-respiratory system, whilst increasing our metabolic rate.

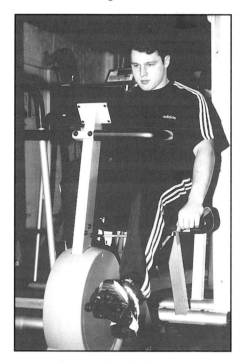

Aerobic activity, improves the shape your heart is in and this is no longer in question. In addition, weight control, stress reduction, toning the body and fat control are also bi-products of aerobic activity, which in summary, are :-

1. **Burns off excess calories.**
2. **Increases the body's ability to burn fat efficiently.**
3. **Lowers your body fat 'set point'.**
4. **Allows you to increase your calorific intake so as to be able to build muscle mass whilst losing fat.**

Recumbent Bike - it better separates the use of legs and body and prevents the 'rolling' action which can occur in the normal stationary bike when the going gets hard. You can train for both muscle and cardio endurance.

Endurance activities have a different effect on muscle size in that they increase the ability of the body to burn fat by increasing the number and density of 'mito-chondria', which are the 'energy factors' in the cells.

We talk about 'stroke volume' in **Chapter 3 - 'The Human Machine',** which is the amount of blood pumped during each beat. Aerobic exercise trains your heart so it grows. It's pumping chambers enlarge so, as we know, it is able to pump more blood with each beat. You have to stress the heart to make it more efficient and, broadly, we are told that this level of stress needs to be approximately, when training, at a level of 60-80% of the hearts maximum capacity.
This should be the perfect aerobic level at which to work (for a well trained individual, this range may be more appropriate at 70 - 90%).

For example take a male aged 30, the way to work out the ideal heart rate band is to subtract this age figure from 220.
In this case this gives us a figure to work with of 190.
From this subtract the resting heart rate - say- 60 gives us a figure of 130. This figure is referred to as your 'heart rate reserve'.
Work out your percentage, in this case, say 70%, giving 91.
Add back the resting rate we deducted before, giving us a TARGET RATE of 151.
Keep within 5 beats of this, with steady work. This is not a formula for working with weights as bursts of effort are brought into play.

A simpler way is to simply subtract your age from 220 and keep your heart rate again between the 70-90% range - assuming, as we did above, that you are a well trained person.

You must, however, always be attempting to push back you aerobic capacity. This is known as the 'Threshold Pace' or the threshold speed at which you start some Anaerobic respiration.

As you will learn from the chapter on Nutrition, the body is always metabolising protein (aminos), carbs (in the form of glucose and glycogen stored in the cells and liver) and fat in some combination and we can alter that combination of these elements that the body draws on for energy. For example, during the first 35 minutes of aerobic exercise, regardless of intensity, your body draws upon and metabolises primarily carbohydrates. Thereafter and depending upon the body's makeup, you draw on fat reserves.

Cardiovascular Density

This refers to the size and number of blood vessels in a muscle. These blood vessels carry oxygen and nutrients to the muscles cells and, as we know, transport waste products away. Our muscles are limited in size by the amount of nutrients they receive.

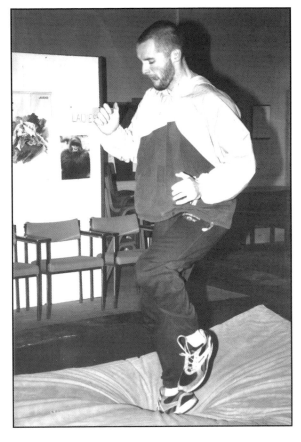

Tony Sykes - running on the spot on the 'crash mat'. It doesn't take very long before you reach the anaerobic threshold.

The more blood vessels you create and the better your cardiovascular density, the more nutrients can be supplied. Blood vessels are an important component in recovery and growth.

Aerobics also increases blood supply to the muscles and builds important blood pathways - more blood, more 'pump', more growth. Aerobics create new, longer blood routes, giving the facility for both more intense and longer workouts. Aerobics also allows faster recovery, as you create greater muscle endurance, which is the capacity of your muscles to continue contracting without fatigue.

Also we develop a greater ability to better utilise oxygen. Cardiovascular conditioning gives us more energy and endurance, better facilitates the removal of toxins and waste products, gives better recovery, less rest between sets, better recovery after a workout and lessens the risk of heart and lung diseases. Aerobic activity is a great metabolic activator - it stimulates our metabolism and will eventually burn fat for energy.

Breathing

My advise to you in this regard is do it!. After that I'm of no help whatsoever. I've never been able to analyse properly how I breath during various types of training, so I haven't a clue as to how

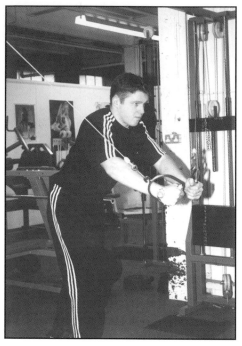

Cable Crossovers - can be used for high reps with medium weight, to build muscle endurance or heavy, as a basic, size building exercise.

anyone should go about it. Whether you should breathe through your nose, mouth or mouth and nose seems a semantic argument. When you need air you'd breathe through your arse if you could. Just get it in.

General Circuit Training

Circuit Training these days, has come to mean anything that rotates a variety of training exercises (stances), in a 40-60 minute programme, which can be based around any primary sport or cross-training exercise. Routines ie. a 'circuit' can be constructed around a boxercise session or a step session or even a weights session and broadly we seek to activate 3 things with any circuit.

1. **Aerobic fitness.**
2. **Muscular endurance.**
3. **Muscular strength.**

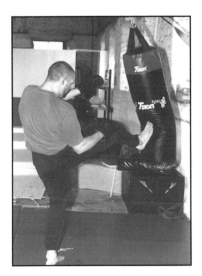

Bag work, wind sprints and free weights can all be mixed together for combat cross-training.

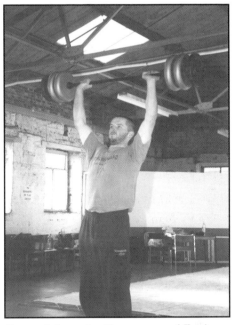

Sets to failure of military press - following a hard Karate session. This is hard cross training for combat.

1. Aerobics - seek to place moderate to heavy loads on the aerobic system for 20 minutes +. Different stations on the circuit can place different levels of effort, with own body resistance and weight resistance being used only to a moderate level.

2. Muscular endurance - will play greater demands on the body at each station and will place much more emphasis on working a muscle group to failure over a 'rep' range of 15 - 30 reps.

3. Muscular strength - will require overloading the muscles so as to achieve failure at the 6 - 10 rep range and require a full minute's recovery between sets.

Such innovations as the 'PACE' gyms, where the circuit is built around resistance equipment, can be 'all things to all people'. But we can design our own circuits very simply and to suit our specific requirements. For combat we need to make a compromise with the endurance/strength components. In attempting to achieve these, we also, over the period of the various exercises, enhance our cardio-vascular capacity. More later ......

Aerobic Equipment

These come in the guise of treadmills, rowers, steppers, climbers, and variations on a theme such as recumbent bikes for example. I use them all and they are an effective way of ensuring a continuing aerobic capacity. Used constructively they can also be used to enhance muscular strength, endurance and anaerobic tolerance.

The treadmill still comes out top in comparative tests on the various machines effectiveness at burning calories. Tests conducted at Wisconsin University showed that at three levels of effort, hard, moderate and light the treadmill still 'burnt' more calories per hour than all the other equipment. At the hard level the treadmill topped 850 cals, compared with 700 for the stepper, 700 for the rower and 600 for the bike.

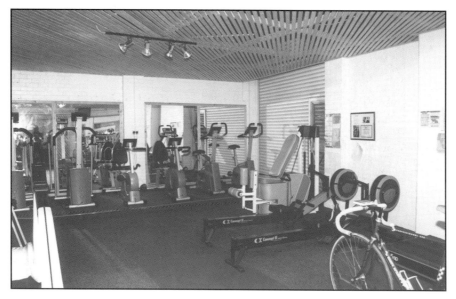

A good CV room, attached to a comprehensive weights gym, which is ideal - (Sporting Bodies - Wakefield, West Yorkshire).

Cross-Training

Everything we talk about in this book, is essentially geared towards 'cross-training'. The object is to produce - by encompassing all aspects of the training overload - Athleticism, Muscularity and Fitness.

In cross-training we hope to effect both our slow-twitch type 1 muscle fibers, by long, slow aerobic conditioning and our fast-twitch type 2 fibers, which, unlike the former, have a high level of myosin ATPase, hence the shorter contraction time. We require in '**combative fitness**' to *power cross-train.* High speed, ballistic movement, even sometimes applied to weights, all contribute to our power potential. It is also thought that high speed, high velocity movements, carry over to be of benefit in 'low speed' aerobic work.

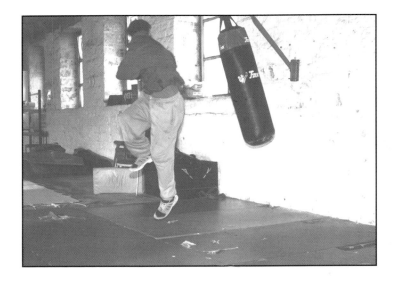

Bob Sykes coming back down after the spinning back kick. An example of power, timing, accuracy, flexibility, but more importantly - practice.

By cross-training, we also allow heavily worked muscle groups to rest properly and also achieve positive adaptation. Our main goal should be to maintain athleticism, which is one of the aspects that can be lost if concentration is solely based on one singular training aspect, such as weights. Flexibility - gained through good stretching and the result of other complex movements, contributes greatly to injury prevention. Cross-training is also thought to beneficially enhance what is scientifically called 'neuromuscular adaption'. Put simply, by constantly changing sports and exercises, you may enhance motor control and muscular efficiency.

Plyometrics

This is essentially playing on the body's protective 'stretch-reflex' mechanism, to improve a muscle's ability to store elastic energy and is also encompassed in our combative training. Essentially a product of the former Soviet-Bloc training routines it was seized upon over here some years back as the Holy Grail, to improve athletic performance. It does, but only in those sports which would benefit from an improved vertical or lateral explosiveness. As we have said elsewhere Plyometric exercises assist in the development of muscles ability to store 'kinetic energy'.

In many ways using plyometrics could possibly be a better way to develop 'power' than weights which tend to generate what is known as 'gross' strength. We're told plyometrics can produce a 5% increase in speed and a 10% improvement in vertical jumping. Repetitions are a big influence on the effectiveness of plyos. Ideally single plyo exercises develop the maximum loading potential, whereas such things as skipping water down effectiveness as they really only lead to muscular endurance.

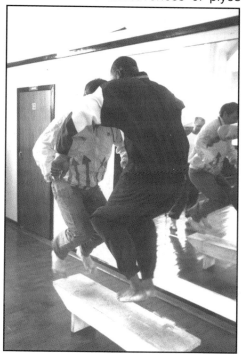

Plyos can be used to develop dynamic power in the arms, legs, and torso, but they should only be done alongside a good weights programme. Muscles, tendons and ligaments all need to be strong in the first place before you should attempt any deep plyometric jumps such as depth jumps. You can include 'bounding' into your sprint work or general running work, which is an excellent way to build leg power. It's not easy, as the landing needs to be made flat footed. The leg is held more

Bench jumps - one minute and you will probably have reached a painful threshold for ankles and calves.

rigid than in running and should be done for some 20 paces.

Warming Up & Stretching

The first thing you should be told is that you should! However, to be perfectly honest, I am one of the worst 'warmers up' going - it must be a boredom thing. The sequence should be:

Warm Up & Stretch Out

For years, in Karate, it was just the opposite, with highly dynamic and ballistic stretching, performed without the benefit of warmed up muscles and increased blood flow.

The warm up should be light and very aerobic, either jogging on the spot, light skipping, easy jogging around the gym or very relaxed shadow boxing - no kicking. To get joints, tendons, muscles and connective tissue properly warmed up, takes about 5 minutes. At that point you can start to stretch out, but don't make it too ballistic ie. lunging up and down on a hamstring stretch etc. After 3 minutes of stretching, jog around again, skip or move so as to 'shake things out' and then stretch again. This is now commonly referred to as 'pre-activity' or 'the low level aerobic activity phase'.

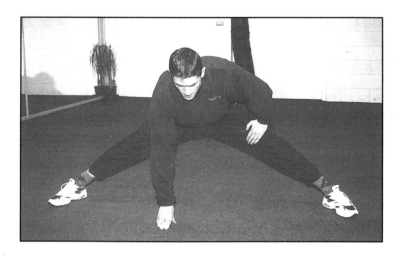

Stretch slowly and carefully and avoid any ballistic movements. Hold each stretch and come up carefully.

You may decide to combine your warm-up with your full CV session of 20 - 30 mins, or whatever, by keeping the first 5 minutes at low intensity. This is okay, but the problem then is that you move into the increased effort phase with no stretching. This is a particular problem when on CV machines.

We need the pre-activity to warm the blood and muscles. Warm muscles are less prone to being 'pulled' than cold ones. The increased warm blood supply to the muscles also affects the surrounding ligaments and tendons and allows the muscle, when it starts to work, to contract in a more efficient way. Also, there will be an increased amount of oxygen in the tissue for increased performance capability.

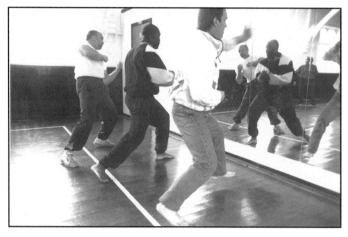

Medium paced shadow boxing (no kicking) is a good warm-up prior to stretching out.

Make the stretching specific to what you're going to do. For example, I won't spend too long on stretching my legs if all I'm going to do is hand work on the bag, but I'll still stretch them. If, however, I'm going to sprint, then I know I'll pull muscles if I'm not warmed up and stretched out prior to hitting the hill. The beauty of hill work, as a side issue, is that is removes the heavy pounding your body takes on the flat, but you use more effort in 'pulling' and 'pushing' on a hill, even your arms, which have a far greater swinging motion. It's very easy to pull some very deep muscles, particularly in the glutes and hamstrings.

I know that increased flexibility helps in the prevention of injuries during training. Some basic stretching exercises are shown in this book, but you should find stretching exercises which suit you. Stretch to a point just reaching discomfort and hold - don't bounce. Slowly release the tension and try again. When you've trained in flexibility for some years, you know your own 'flexibility groove'. When you're warmed up, and start to stretch, you know whether, that day, you are stiffer than usual or whether one leg is more reluctant to reach its optimum flexibility than you are familiar with. With this inner feeling, you are usually able to 'favour' a part of your body which is not properly loosened up, but to achieve this somewhat nirvanic state, where you know your body that well, may take years.

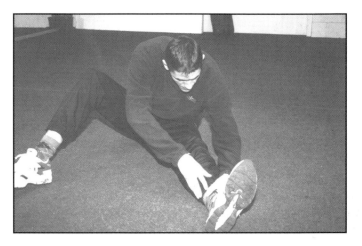

PNF stretching. When you reach your maximum stretch, apply muscular force with the leg as if you were trying to force your heel into the ground. Relax, come off the stretch and then stretch again, hopefully, now with a lower stretch. In this particular stretch, always stretch your chest to your leg, not your head

Stretching can be broadly one of three types, bouncing or ballistic, stationary or static, and thirdly, **PNF** (proprioceptive neuromuscular facilitation), stretch. For many years in martial arts, we were subjected to a wild and dangerous variety of ballistic stretching, including ballistically assisted stretches with partners, which practice, fortunately, has now been accepted as unsound. The static stretch, on the other hand, is often exactly the same stretch, but with a consistent force placed against the stretch.

The PNF stretch, originally designed to help in rehabilitation of patients with partial paralysis, is somewhat of an advance on the basic static stretch, but asks that as we reach the extent of the stretch, that we exert some pressure into the stretch which fools our nerve endings into thinking there is more load being exerted than there actually is. The next stretch we do should then have more movement in it.

When you achieve good flexibility, you'll find yourself at all times of the day, clicking, stretching, rotating and pulling parts of your body. I do it with my back, wrists, neck, shoulders and ankles all the time, and most of it is involuntary. I'll also stretch my hamstrings from a seated position, and, much to the annoyance of Dawn, my better half, rotate my back until it clicks and also click all my fingers.

Overtraining

If training is good - is more better?

Over-training starts with fatigue. Fatigue, as we will see in Chapter 3, is defined by scientists as *"failure to maintain a specified force or power output"*. What we didn't say in the chapter on 'The Human Machine' is that it's purpose is to protect our bodies and it's muscles from serious damage caused by extreme exertion.

We're told that fatigue is a subjective sensation, with it's routines in the metabolic, circulatory and nervous system changes that occur during physical stress. The result is that you get physically and mentally weaker.

Chapter 3 - 'The Human Machine', looks at the depletion and accumulation theories. Waste products in your tissues from excess exercise include: lactic, pyruvic and sucinic acids, ammonia and urea. All this is balanced against the depletion of fuel stores such as key minerals and electrolytes and the chemicals that carry messages. Waste build-up interferes with your production of energy and also inhibits the muscles ability to contract and relax.

Overtraining also causes more problems through injuries, decrease of maximum performance, decrease of maximum power output and decrease of maximum strength. Weight loss and flu-like symptoms can also occur. The body's defence mechanism is to decrease performance or 'shut down' when the capacity to adapt to training demands is exceeded. Quantity and duration are more critical factors than the type of training performed.

On the mental side, it is thought that ammonia build-up also has a detrimental effect on the concentration of neurotransmitters in the brain. On top of all this, acids and ammonia begin to interfere with the breakdown of the high-energy phosphates that your body uses in large quantities during intense exercise.

We are also told that fatigue produces a leakage of potassium from the fibers of the muscles. Potassium is critical to the responsiveness, contraction capabilities and endurance of the muscle cells themselves. As potassium supplies diminish, so do strength and endurance. Adequate time must be allowed for recovery from a hard workout and to replenish energy stores. It is believed that the fast twitch, speed orientated muscles need more time to recover than the slow twitch, endurance ones. Bigger muscles also need longer. Its a fairly obvious point to make, but high intensity effort, requires a longer recovery period than moderate effort.

Stress, poor diet and injury, all add to recovery time. You should know yourself well enough to be able to measure heart rate recovery, breathing recovery and appetite recovery. Being tired, irritable, having a poor sleep pattern and other problems can all be symptomatic of overtraining. It also has an eventual **catabolic** effect ie. breakdown of muscle tissue.

Most training is **anabolic** ie. it causes muscles to grow. The flipside of this is that exercise, even weight lifting is also catabolic - as we have said, the process by which your muscles lose mass. High intensity training heightens our body's catabolic responses, particularly the production of cortisol. Cortisol is one of the body's most potent catabolic hormones. Apart from ensuring we don't overtrain, what is required, as we outline in the chapter on Nutrition, is to ensure the equality by the addition of some nutritional advantage.

Stress

Although not specifically of significance to training for combat, training for 'stress release' should have a mention. Conflict and possible physical confrontation are often manifestations of gross over-reaction to situations which, if analysed in the cold light of day, by rational people, would appear to be irrational acts - 'road rage', 'trolley rage' not being the least of these - seemingly. The pace of today's lifestyle is highly stressful. Uncertainty of work prospects, competition, increased volumes of traffic and attendant frustration, being bombarded daily by sounds and sensations, that even 15 years ago were considerably less, all contribute to a build-up of stress that can have damaging physical and psychological effects.

One resultant problem is that the body can be in a constant state of muscle tension - this has been referred to as 'baseline tension'. Hamstrings, neck and back muscles all may have a high level of baseline tension, together with a stiffening of the diaphragm. The latter can lead to both breathing deficiencies and digestive problems, with hyper-ventilation often leading to high blood pressure. Also the increased heart rate and muscle tension in arteries, can result in permanently raised blood pressure and heart strain.

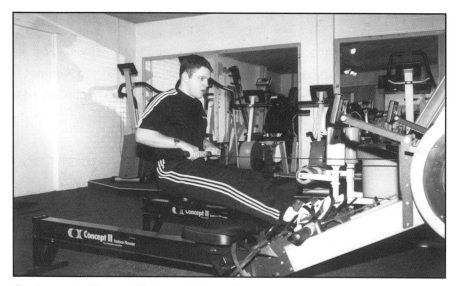

Rowing on the 'Concept II'. One of the best all-round pieces of CV equipment. By increasing the resistance and intensity of effort, it will also produce good muscle endurance.

If blood is pumped through the body at abnormally high pressures this gives rise to the condition known as high blood pressure. A normal resting pressure is 120/80, whereas someone with high blood pressure may measure 140/90. Such long term, pressures can cause damage to the heart, kidneys and the blood vessels themselves. This is a thickening known as ateriosclerosis. Excessive blood fats accumulate in the suffering arteries and if the coronary arteries become obstructed, depriving the heart muscle of oxygen, then a heart attack may occur. Also decreased blood flow to the kidneys results in a failure of the kidneys to remove impurities from the blood, resulting in the accumulation of high toxic wastes in the body. There is also the possibility of strokes since it can cause a clot or fragment of artheriosclerotic plaque that blocks the blood flow to break free and flow to the brain.

One particular type of heart rate has nothing to do with physical exercise and its called the 'anticipatory' or 'tension' rate and its the emotional heart rate. This is usually in response to both mental and physical stimulae and prepares us, partly, for the flight or fight syndrome, pumping blood and oxygen around the body, even before you've made a move. In situations of acute emotional stress, the sympathetic nervous system, that is the automatic system that speeds up most of the body's activities, combines with the output of the adrenal glands, to produce a high level of hormones in the blood, which when they reach the heart, cause it to increase in rate and strength of contraction. As a point of interest, this is usually contrasted by the **Parasympathetic System,** which acts as a damper - to keep the hormone effect down to safe levels.

Stomach ulcers, heartburn and other internal problems, result from a poor blood supply to the gut. Stress, over a long period, has the effect of triggering our body's **sympathetic nervous system.** Adrenaline, released from nerve endings, triggers the 'fight or flight' responses such as raised heart rate, raised blood pressure, blood directed away from internal organs to the musculature and shallow, tense breathing. All this is fine if we are about to fight or flight so to speak, but it is seriously detrimental if all we are doing is fighting our way through more traffic chaos or opening the mail at our desk. Add to all this, a long-term suppression of our immune system and you can see why stress is a killer.

Without the release that exercise gives us, a 'bottling up' takes place, to be eventually released irrationally and inappropriately in other situations - in the street, in the pub or club, in the home and on the road, as tempers fly. A high resting heart rate in the 70s or 80s can indicate a stressed body. Training is the balance on life and as the pace increases, we need it more not less. We need to be in control of ourselves and often, we are the last people to recognise irrational and unstable behaviour. Avoidance of conflict is paramount and seeing a situation incorrectly, is a sign we are letting stress take a hold.

Training and the Immune System

The Immune System, is composed of white cells in the blood and other specialised tissues such as the Lymph Nodes. When exposed to an invading substance, the body mounts a defense, such as the B Lymphocytes that produce anti-bodies to neutralise foreign invaders. Lymphocytes also produce long-term immunity.

When attacked, they, hopefully, overcome the invading force and with their 'immunalogical memory', which programmes them to always defeat quickly that same invading force. Therefore, simulation has the same effect, that is immunisation re exposure to a non-virulant form of the micro-organism eg. smallpox, tetanus, polio etc etc. The effectiveness reaches peak maturity at 16 -18 years then declines.

It is understood, that exercise helps keep our immune system in fighting shape. Clinical studies would seem to have proved how exercise helps by possibly an increasing number of lymphocytes - particularly in older people, whose immune system is on the way out.

However, the other side of the coin is that studies have shown that over-training can decrease immunity. High intensity, highly strenuous sports, can cause a seeming increase in infections, particularly respiratory ones and the probable cause would seem to be stress. Heavy, taxing workouts without sufficient recovery time, cause stress and stress is a known 'immunosuppressor'. The hormone 'cortisol' is released when stress is present, which is not only catabolic, with regard to the negative effect on muscles, but also suppresses the immune system.

Adrenal hormones are also released under stress. There are other factors at work, but I can personally support the over-training theory. During those periods when I've done too much for too long, I'll come down with a more or less permanent cold, throat infection or bad chest - fit, but knackered! I know that it's been due to overtraining and that my body is somehow out of sync.

Heat in Training

Some years ago, a former University student and athletic blue, suffered severe injuries as a result of running in an 8 km race, which had been cancelled by the race organisers due to the extreme heat - some 40 degrees centigrade. The result was an extreme case of Rhabdomyolysis, caused by severe dehydration and the onset of heat stroke. He suffered the amputation of a leg, kidney failure and some CNS damage.

Thermo-Regulation

As humans, we are classed as Homiotherms ie. our body temperature remains reasonably constant, regardless of the external environment. The body's core temperature is in dynamic equilibrium at all times and if it varies by more than a few degrees, the results can be catastrophic. Survival is about maintaining a constant heat production/heat loss balance, which will maintain the core temperature of the body within those safe limits.

Self-Controlling Mechanism

The body's metabolism is the main source of heat production and even when sleeping, a substantial amount of heat is produced. When exercising, the muscle effect contributes greatly to the heat generated and the metabolic rate can increase by some 20-25 times above base resting levels, which can rapidly and substantially increase core temperature.

The hormones Thyroxine (Thyroid hormone) and Adrenalin, also increase metabolic rate and so, in the heat of 'competition' or 'battle', a very dangerous situation develops, where increased heat can become self-perpetuating.

The body has its own temperature gauge called the 'Hypothalmus', which is a small portion of the brain and reacts to increases in heat by initiating a specific response or activity and increase in the rate of heat dissipation. Heat, of course, from external conditions may also increase the heat which is being internally generated. However, eventually, at extremely high core temperatures, the body's 'thermostat' loses its ability to cope, the internal temperature climbs further and unless extreme action is taken to cool down, the result is a system failure.

The main defence is not to shut down heat production but increase the body's 4 methods of heat dissipation which are:-

1. Radiation - heat transferred out to a, usually, colder environment. This is not a foolproof system, particularly, if the outside is hotter, as the result can be that the process reverses itself.

2. Conduction - essentially, this is 'object to object' ie getting into water or a cold shower.

3. Convection - cold air, moving over the skin causes heat to be lost by convection as the layer of warm air near the skin is moved away.

4. Evaporation - this process, accounts for our body's major physiological defence against overheating. We are told, that we have some 3 million sweat glands distributed over the body's surface. In it's defence, the body sweats and the evaporation provides a cooling effect. The cooled skin, in turn, cools the blood which returns to the body's core.

When the ambient air temperature is very high, effective cooling by means other than evaporation is markedly decreased and so evaporation can remain the only effective method. Humidity is also a critical factor in determining how even that remains an effective means of cooling. If sweat forms, but does not evaporate, it stays or just falls off, which is a dangerous situation, as it is not the process of sweating which cools but the process of that sweat evaporating. A bad situation exists when high temperatures are combined with high humidity.

The circulatory system ie. the blood supply, is all important in retaining thermal balance. Blood is pumped out to the periphery, where arteries and veins dilate, to enhance radiative heat loss. This is why you get reddened or flushed during exercise, particularly on a hot day. Given favourable external circumstances, cooled blood returns to internal areas, picks up more heat to transfer to outer layers.

Sweating begins very early during exercise and reaches equilibrium in about half an hour, depending upon exercise intensity. Hormonal action is important, as water and electrolytes are lost in the process of sweating. The pituatory gland (a small but vital organ in the brain), releases a hormone called 'anti diuretic hormone' (ADH). This tells the kidneys to increase water absorption. How yellow your urine is after a bout of heavy exercise, indicates that it contains less water and is more concentrated. Another hormone 'Aldosterone' is released which helps conserve sodium, also lost in the sweating process.

Also, during long exercise, the amount of blood pumped throughout the body has to remain constant, so less is shunted to the periphery, so as to maintain cardiac output. Blood is also diverted away from digestive tissues and to the muscles. It would seem, we are told, that in hot conditions, work is accomplished more by anaerobic metabolism leading to an early accumulation of lactic acid.

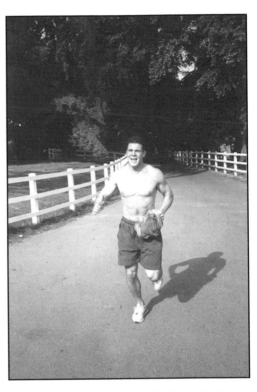

Coming in first on a summer Bodyguard selection course. Only a short run in this case, but if the run was of any distance, heat would be a problem.

Clothes in hot conditions should be light, airy and, depending on your dress preference, white in colour. Dark or black clothing absorbs heat and adds to radiation heat gain. Don't change into dry clothes, as sweat soaked wet clothes, promote evaporation. One statistic I saw was that in America they have attributed 70 footballing deaths to heat stroke in 23 years. We never do it, but we are told to acclimatise the body over about a one week period.

Trained people benefit by having a better adaptation to the physiological requirements of sweating than do unfit ones and this has been shown to be particularly noticeable in older people.

Heat stress can be fatal and characterised by thirst, unsteadiness, extreme fatigue and visual disturbance. In all cases where heat is becoming a problem, one should cease exercise and rehydrate.

Heat cramps - a mild form of physical problems caused by heat, but none the less, a warning sign along the way. Again, cease exercise and take water, together with electrolytes.

Heat exhaustion - identified by a weak, rapid pulse, dizziness, headache and nausea and is usually a problem for untrained people who have ineffective circulatory adjustments and excess sweating, which depletes blood volume, often not replaced by adequate water intake. The treatment should be the removal to a cooler environment and large amounts of fluid. It should be remembered that for the body to retain a good circulatory efficiency, the blood requires a high fluid content and oversweating reduces this, and as a consequence the blood's viscosity.

Heat stroke - the complete failure of the heat regulatory mechanisms of the body. It requires immediate medical attention and delay can be fatal. Sweating usually ceases and the skin becomes dry and hot and consequently, the body temperature rises to dangerous levels, with a circulatory collapse. Immerse in cold water or ice packs.

Regular trainers should ensure that they replace the minerals lost in sweating such as zinc, copper, manganese and trace elements. Deficiencies can occur over long periods.

Training Injuries

With the best preparation, careful stretching, adequate nutrition we will still injure ourselves, particularly if we engage in combative pastimes as well. When injured the sensible advise is to seek professional help. I never do, but the common sense approach should be to seek assistance from someone who knows. Usually this isn't in the shape of your GP, although they have got better over the years, as the usual direction has been, for many years, to "rest it' for a few weeks. I'm of the self-help school of medicine and with self-massage, care and carefully working the injury you can, with most things, get the damaged part back into shape.

Physiotherapists, Chiropractors, Acupuncturists, Sports Masseurs etc, these days, are usually well-trained and well versed in a range of therapy that usually allows training to continue during recovery of a particular injury. It is only over the past few years that Western medicine has taken a more pragmatic and common sense approach to sports injuries.

Overview

Moderate intensity - 50%-60% of max. (a level of effort for someone starting out)
Fat Burning - 60%-70% of max.
Good Fitness Gains - 70%-80% of max.
Performance Enhancement - 80%-100% . At more than 100% you will become anaerobic and then your system will start to shut down due to Lactic acid build-up.

Calorie Burn

Various exercises have a greater potential to burn calories. For the following short list of various types of exercise, the calories burned per minute by a 170lb (70 kilos) man are roughly:

Running (7mph or 3.1m/s)	-	15.5 calories
Skipping (120 turns per minute)	-	14.8 calories
Boxing (sparring)	-	12.1 calories
Circuit Training	-	10.8 calories
Bodybuilding/weight training	-	8 calories
Walking (4mph)	-	5.4 calories

CHAPTER 3

THE HUMAN MACHINE

To understand the science of fitness, training and diet we need to know something about what makes us tick. I've divided the subject matter into various sections - in no order of importance. There can't be any order as each aspect is equally as important. Apologies for any long words, but I didn't make them up and in describing how a thing works it's pretty much impossible to without resorting to the technical phrase where appropriate. It has been said earlier that this book is not about psychology, and equally it is not about human biology or the science of nutrition, however, without a working knowledge you are training in the dark. You must know how your body functions so as to get the best out of yourself or correct under-performance. I think it's a true statement that most people who train know how the internal combustion engine works far better than they know how they, themselves work.

WHAT IS LIFE ?? - Life is very simply about having an *oxygenated blood supply'.*

The Lungs

It all starts here, where oxygen from the air is extracted via the millions of tiny air sacs ie the Alveoli, around which the blood flows . Atmospheric pressure forces the oxygen onto the sacs which are like balloons dangling in the liquid of your blood-stream. Then following the 'law of gaseous diffusion', the oxygen moves from the area of high pressure in the Alveoli to the red blood cells, where the pressure is lower. The red blood cells are like empty bottles at this stage having given up returning wastes which we have breathed out, such as carbon dioxide and water, exchanged in the muscles and organs for the oxygen, which the red blood cells have given up. How effective the exchange is, is limited by the number of red blood cells and the haemoglobin they carry, even if the lungs could process more oxygen.

This 'oxygenated' blood supply is then pumped around the body by the action of the heart to the vital organs, in particular the brain and muscles. It eventually leaves the arteries via capillaries with porous walls which allows the oxygen to permeate into the organs. The veins take the de-oxygenated blood and waste gases back to the lungs where we expel them as we breathe.

What about our oxygen processing capacity. Broadly with 21% of oxygen in air, the balance being nitrogen, we manage to process some 7% only. The lungs have no muscles of their own, it is the muscles in the ribcage which expand and contract.

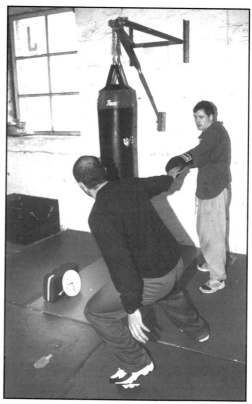

When we move to some sort of action, there are two limiting factors to capacity, Ie, the size of the vacuum your muscles create for your lungs to expand into and, secondly, the size of the area they can be squeezed back into. A well conditioned man, as he moves into action, has the capability for inhaling more air and for longer periods and, for exhaling more waste because the muscles in the chest are trained to do more work.

Wind sprints, against the clock, can often cause too much demand for oxygen that cannot be processed and anaerobic tolerance is then required.

This is limited by the condition of the muscles surrounding the lungs.

The second major limiting factor on how much air your lungs can process is the condition inside them. Lungs also vary in size, usually in relation to body size. In sport, we are less concerned with size, more with how much of the total lung capacity is usable. This usable portion is called 'Vital Capacity' and can be measured in the laboratory by the amount of air that can exhaled in one deep breath. A 'well conditioned' male's Vital Capacity is approx. 75% of his total lung capacity. Often, however, an unfit man can match this, so we must look at one more test which is the Maximum Minute Volume and is actually the amount of air you can process in one minute and separates the men from the boys. Again, a well conditioned man will force as much as 20 times his Vital Capacity through his lungs in one minute, whilst an 'out-of-condition' man will be hard pressed to force even 10 times through. He simply lacks the muscles and strength to achieve.

The remainder of the air in your lungs, after the usable lung volume has been measured, is called the 'Residual Volume', which volume is fixed and even a fit man can't breath it in or out. With no exercise, the Residual Volume increases, whilst with training, there will be an increase in both muscle ability and usable volume.

At rest, the oxygen supplied to the blood is only about 1 cup per minute. Extreme exercise, in a well trained athlete, can step this up to as much as 1 gallon per minute. At rest, only about 12% of the stagnant air in the lungs is renewed during each breath.

A good way to test the breathing condition of your lungs is to take a deep breath and hold it. Most adults in moderately good physical condition and with healthy lungs, should be able to hold their breath for a minute or longer.

Heart

This keeps the whole assembly line going. As we know, it takes oxygen-laden blood from the lungs, pumps it throughout the body and takes carbon dioxide-laden blood back to the lungs, where it is exchanged for more oxygen. Ironically, the heart works faster and less efficiently when you give it nothing to do. Both anaerobically and aerobically-conditioned males, who exercise regularly, will have a resting heart rate of 60 beats per minute or less. A poorly conditioned man could be 80 or more.

Heart Rate
    Resting

	Normal Person	70 - 80
	Very Athletic	30 - 40
	Good Trainer	50 - 60

    Maximum heart rate for most healthy people under 60 = 155 - 210

If we extrapolate this, a well conditioned man at rest has a heart rate of 3,600 beats per hour, which over 24 hours amounts to 86,400 heartbeats. By contrast, a poorly conditioned man with a resting rate of 4,800 beats per hour over 24 hours has achieved some 115,200, so even at complete rest, a poorly conditioned man who does not exercise has had a heart that has had to beat 30,000 times more each day of his life.

There are 2 main training effects on the heart. Like any muscle, a non-trained heart, is usually small and weak. An enlarged, unhealthy heart can often grow that way to compensate for some deficiency in the cardiovascular system. By contrast, the athlete's heart is strong, healthy, relatively large and highly efficient, pumping more blood with each stroke. Vascularity plays a part, as a healthy heart is well supplied with blood itself.

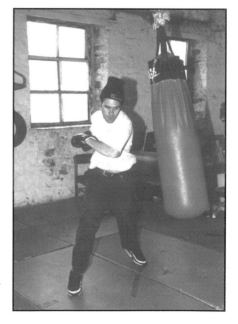

For rounds on the bag, you need a well-functioning heart. Fortunately bag work will give you that.

Healthy hearts work at maximum output - peaking at 190 beats per minute, whilst poorly conditioned hearts go as high as 220. Some supremely well conditioned athletes, who are run to exhaustion on treadmills, have never reached beyond 165-170 beats per minute. Well conditioned hearts can do twice as much, run twice as fast or twice as long. As an example of an extreme sport, cross-country skiers can hold their hearts at 170 bpm for up to 2.5 hours.

Stroke Volume

This is the term used to describe how much blood is pushed out of the left ventricle with each beat. One very important element in the overall training effect is your heart's stroke volume, because the more you pump out with each beat, the fewer times your heart will be required to beat. There is a thing called the 'Ejection Fraction' and a well trained person can push about 95% of blood in the left ventricle, whilst working at 80%. The average untrained person, pushes only 75% whilst working at 80%. Remember - that blood is going to your working muscles and organs and how effectively the oxygen it's carrying gets there and is taken into the muscle cells and utilised, is called your MAX VO_2 uptake. Highly trained marathon runners and cross-country skiers have been known to have MAX VO_2 uptake in excess of 75 millilitres of oxygen per kilo of bodyweight, per minute! That's compared to the sedentary person who only uses 40ml/kilo/min.

So training benefits the heart in several ways - developing it into a strong healthy muscle that works more effortlessly, either during moments of relaxation or during peak physical exertion and by doing so, maintaining large reserves of power to handle whatever physical or emotional stress is placed on it.

Blood

Above, we looked at how, having an 'oxygenated' blood supply is the meaning of life. At rest, blood flows through the arteries at approx. 55 feet per minute. By speeding up the circulation to up to 2-3 times, the same blood volume can be made to do 2-3 times the work of feeding the cells and removing waste. Muscular activity speeds up the normal heart rate, forcing it to pump more blood per minute. The benefits increase manifold. As the volume of blood increases, so does the blood supply to the muscles and this improved blood flow, resulting from tissue 'vascularisation', is probably the most remarkable phenomenon of the training effect. Newer and smaller routes open up due to the demands.

Vessels enlarge and increase in number as an adaptive response to training demand. Also, the fat metabolism, particularly of cholesterol, a naturally produced product in the body, but also ingested in fats, which can clog the arterial walls and hardens the arteries. Essentially, training flushes this away.

The training effect produces more blood, specifically more red blood cells that carry the haemoglobin, more blood plasma that carries the red blood cells and consequently, more total blood volume. An average sized man may increase his blood volume by nearly a quart in response to aerobic conditioning.

The blood cell count increases proportionately. This gives both a greater oxygen carrying capacity and more capacity to remove

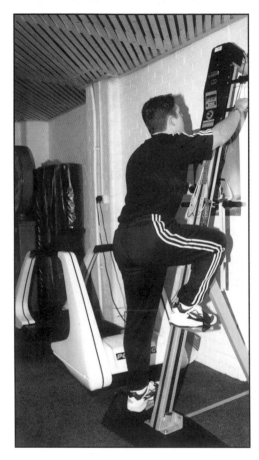

The Versa-Climber. Probably one of the most demanding of CV equipment. Without practice and conditioning, it is very easy to go anaerobic.

wastes. The removal of carbon dioxide and other waste products is just as important in reducing fatigue and increasing endurance, as is, the production of energy.

Training does 3 things to blood vessels:-

1. Enlarges them and makes them more pliable to pressure.

2. Increases their number for saturation coverage.

3. Helps keep their linings clear of unwanted materials.

The Tissue

The process of 'Osmosis' is that by which oxygen and food particles, now in liquid form, pass through the cell membrane and waste products exit the cell in the opposite direction. This is life as we know it and its capacity and efficiency increases in proportion to the amount of exercise - the more we demand, the better it will work.

The tissues at the end of the assembly line can be bone, muscle, organ and nerves, the smallest units being individual cells. Each cell is like a small factory with its own goods in and out facility, store room, power plant for creating energy, heat and re-generation. All the oxygen we breathe and food we digest eventually arrives at these cells. The ratio of oxygen to food is critical and if there is too much food, the store room fills up.

Cells build up to make tissue such as bone, muscle and nerves - various tissues combine to form organs such as heart, lungs and digestive organs. Several organs combine to form entire systems such as the Pulmonary and Cardiovascular systems.

The Central Nervous System (CNS)

Essentially comprised of the Brain and Spinal Cord, the CNS receives signals and after interpreting them sends them back. The Peripheral Nervous System is the part which relays messages from the main CNS to the body (called the Efferent system) and relays messages the other way from the body to the CNS (called the Offerent system). It gets somewhat complicated as the efferent system ie the system designed to cause action' is itself divided into two parts - the Somantic system, which is designed for voluntary actions and the Autonomic system, which processes and activates involuntary action eg breathing.

The Offerent system which sends messages to the CNS receives messages from three different types of receptors

1. **Proprioceptors** - located in the joints, muscle tendons and the inner ear are responsible for detecting the bodies position and movement.

2. **Exteroceptors** - located near the skin surface and detect information from outside the body eg sight, touch, heat etc

3 **Enteroceptors** - located in the blood vessels and viscera, they report inner sensations eg hangover, pain, thirst, pressure, fatigue and nausea.

After all that, what if anything, can we do about matters. Well, surprisingly we can alter our CNS to our advantage. If we want greater strength, better pain management, all are modifiable in some way. Strength is very much controlled by the mind. When we weight train, muscle contraction is modified by both internal and external stimuli that the CNS interprets on the basis of a built-in 'self defence' mechanism in the muscle spindles and Golgi Tendon organs. This latter effects how supple we are and we can deceive the golgi tendons during stretching exercises by the application of some effort when in the stretch to increase our flexibility - for example.

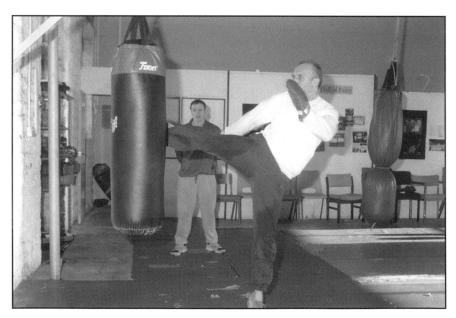

Practice eventually equals co-ordination.

We can, through the excitation of individual motor units in the muscles, alter the threshold level of the golgi tendon organs.

All motor movement is a very complex, time-consuming, re-integration of nervous functions. We have to learn to shut off certain muscles and others to 'turn on', how much 'electro-chemical' charge to send to the muscles , the precise timing involved in literally dozens of sequentially stimulated muscles - The learning process is called PRACTICE and the result is called CO-ORDINATION. Gosh you had to suffer to get to that!

By controlling our minds we can push back the points at which some of our Proprioceptors eg Golgi tendons and muscle spindles are stimulated to inhibit further work - which of course we don't want. The shutdown is the body's self-defence mechanism. It stops us ripping ourselves apart, however they are conservatively metered in that we usually have a lot left.

Most injuries with weights occur through the following
1. Overtraining - 'cumulative microtrauma'
2. Overstraining tissue from exaggerated amplitude
3. Initially overstretched explosive application of effort = kinetic energy

NB over-zealous or exaggerated amplitude is a fancy way of saying - overstretching

Hormones
   Endocrine System
Hormones are secreted by various glands that comprise the Endocrine system. There are two types of hormones -Steroids & Polypeptides

As human beings we are captive to hormones. Everything we eat and every act we do is modified in some way by some hormonal interaction. Hormones regulate almost all our bodily functions. They regulate growth and development, help cope with physical and mental stress and regulate all forms of training responses, including protein metabolism, fat metabolism and energy production. It should be noted that the CNS and Endocrine system are inseparable - responses from one produce an effect on the other.

Steroid hormones are from cholesterol in the gonads and cerebral core and Polypeptides are manufactured in many other glands from various amino acid combinations.

Hormones act in three different ways:-
1. Alter the rate of synthesis of your cellular protein
2. Change the rate of enzyme activity or
3. Change the rate of transport of nutrients through the cellwalls.

For example Insulin - a hormone manufactured from the pancreas increases cellular uptake of glucose which in turn causes increased synthesis of muscle glycogen. This leads to a decrease in blood/bone glucose which causes a decrease in insulin production. As a consequence of prolonged workouts this decrease in blood glucose and reduced production of insulin causes an increase in the mobilisation of stored fat   --- all that just to loose a few pounds.!!!

On a serious note there is a more complex hormonal reaction to long workouts with the release of a different type of hormone being released ie Glucagon - this eventually due to the take up of aminos in the liver inhibits muscle growth.

Growth Hormone -released through high intensity training as a result of signals to the Hypothalmus

Thyroid Hormones - the Thyroid or 'Master Gland', which is located in the throat. Caused by 'Thyroid Stimulating Hormone' (TSH) it releases two hormones T4 and T3, for short. T4 raises the metabolic rate in the cells as much as four times. Also Carbohydrate and Fat metabolism are greatly facilitated by Thyroxine.

Adrenal Hormones - Adrenal glands are comprised of two parts ie the 'cortex'

(outer layer) and the medulla' (inner section). Exercise dramatically increases the output of Ephinepherine which in turn causes increased blood flow to working muscles, enhanced cardiac output, the mobilisation of energy substrate, fat metabolism and the general 'gearing up' for stress functions.

NB the hormones are Aldosterone, Cortisol, Epinerol, Noreprine.

Glands of the Body

Glands are, essentially, the organs of vitality. When working in top condition, a trained individual experiences a sense of well-being, rather than feeling sluggish and under the weather. Unfortunately, our glands are susceptible to stress, in the form of worry, fear, anger, depression and if these conditions obtain for long periods, the glands secrete, what can only be termed as poisons into the body.

The pancreas, whilst a familiar term to people - if asked the describe what it's function is, they would probably be at a loss. The main function is the production of insulin and a malfunction causes diabetes. The pancreas is helped in its task by B-complex vitamins, which, if absent, cause starch and carbohydrates to lack the necessary enzymes for digestion, thereby overworking the pancreas and so producing an excess amount of sugar.

The adrenals help create the body's strength by producing hormones, as we have seen earlier, and vitamin C has a part to play in this process. The other glands such as the pituatory, thyroid, parathyroid and others, all in some way need the assistance of vitamins and minerals to function properly.

Food

You might think that any subject concerning food should come in Chapter 4 - 'Nutrition', but the following is really the fundamentals.This is not about nutrition, but about the body's processing of 'fuel' to survive and grow.

Attempting to 'grow' lean muscle also often entails eating, to the degree that we can often put on fat, which is a contradictory process. What we are primarily concerned with here is how the body uses food. What types of food, are covered in Chapter 4.

Metabolic Rate

Energy production in the body, ultimately depends on *biological oxydation,* a bi-product of which is heat. The term 'calorie', by which we use to measure the energy in food and the energy expended through exercise, is a unit of heat!. Metabolic rate can be estimated by measuring how much heat your body is producing. **Base Metabolic Rate (BMR)** is the measure of how much energy the body consumes when you are completely at rest. We are told that this is somewhere in the region of 1,000 calories a day or less. Generally the BMR is higher in men than in women, higher for those with more muscle mass and lower for those with less. We are told, for example, that 30 minutes brisk walking burns off 150 cals, 30 mins over normal terrain on a bike 200, swimming 275 and jogging 370.

Exercise is a very important factor in determining how much heat energy the body produces, as well as how various ingested nutrients will be metabolised in the body. The higher the MR the more calories you burn and the leaner you stay. The MR increases with exercise, but it also remains high after the exercise which is good news. Exercise which increases Heart and Respiration rate and which is sustainable over a reasonable period is the best type of exercise when it comes to boosting MR ie Aerobic exercise.

Aerobic means, 'with oxygen' and is, broadly, any exercise that significantly exercises your heart rate and the delivery of oxygen to your muscles via the circulatory system. If, however the exercise is too great, it is not sustainable and can only be maintained for short periods. Running, swimming, biking, treadmills, rowers, stairclimbers, exercise classes etc,etc,etc are all aerobically utilised by people, but, if work rate increases, all are capable of turning the exercise 'Anaerobic - more later.

One thing to know about food intake is that cutting back too much in the hope of losing weight can have a somewhat counter effect as you'll unduly slow down the MR ie the burn of fat! People who go on crash diets rarely achieve the gains they expect. Eating more small meals in a day stimulates the MR and, strangely, protein stimulates the MR by up to 30%, whilst Carbs, and fats achieve some 10% - in other words some protein with each meal keeps a high MR.

Muscle

Muscle is made of protein and protein is made of nitrogen and is a primary calorie burner. The more you have, then during both rest and exercise, you will burn calories. Be careful cutting back food intake because if by eating less you lose lean mass you aggravate the problem. Also too much aerobic work will burn off lean muscle mass and make the problem even harder. The answer lies in what we consume as distinct from solely volume. It would appear that we burn an extra 30-50 calories per day for every pound of muscle we can add. Don't, however, try and gauge your weight gain progress solely by the scales - as they don't just measure increases in lean muscle mass.

Broadly, muscle is made up of 3 types of cell - Myofibrillar, Mitochondria and Sarcoplasm. All 3 are designed to come into play when different 'demands' are placed on the muscle. If you were to lift to 'failure' over only, say, a 6 rep range, you would stimulate only a partial range of muscle cell, being the Myofibrillar in particular. This is the fiber used for explosive power and strength.

To stimulate the other 2 types of muscle, you will need to come off maximum and put in sets which decrease the weight and increase the rep range - 10-12 to primarily stimulate the Mitochondria, the cell within which **ATP** (adenosine triphosphate) synthesis takes place. Higher reps still, will stimulate the Sarcoplasm or 'Striated' fiber and also help increase vascularity.

While were on the subject lets look more closely at muscles. With over 600 muscles in the body it is a complex arrangement. A good muscle tone is the product of the muscles adaptation to expected stress through, say, weight training.

There are 3 basic types -

    Skeletal

    Cardiac

    Smooth

The Skeletal/muscle system is the heaviest and is essentially within our grasp to control. Cardiac and Smooth, such as the digestive tract are not really under our direct control, although we can influence how efficient and capable these muscle groups become. Out of the 600 muscles, some 435 are skeletal and under our control to varying degrees, with the entire skeletal muscle system having some 250,000 - 300,000 individual muscle fibres. In the average male some 40% of bodyweight comes from skeletal muscle.

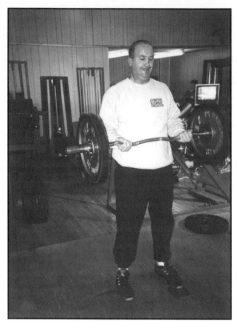

A muscle is composed of millions of compartments of bundles of muscle fibers that help transmit electrical signals for a controlled co-ordinated contraction. Any particular skeletal muscle is comprised of anywhere from 200 large fibres. These fibres are equally composed of several hundred thousand of smaller fibres and at a lower level these are composed of smaller elements

Skeletal muscles we can alter to our own requirements - here, the work is going into the biceps.

called 'Myofibrils'. Further sub-divided and at the root, so to speak, are two smaller elements of contractile protein -Myosin and Actin. Without getting too 'heavy' about how things work what happens is that when a muscle shortens during some movement ('Concentric Contractions' - which is the effort needed to move bones) a 'cross-movement' or 'bridges', takes place between these protein elements.

The signal for the contraction depends upon a nervous impulse strong enough to stimulate the internal mechanism of the muscle which requires the presence of the protein Troponin and Tropomyosin plus minerals Calcium and Magnesium. Muscle contracts in response to an adequate nervous impulse and it is the brain which controls these functions to increase to amazing accuracy.

When a muscle starts to contract, it needs energy to achieve the required result. This energy comes from ATP. ATP consists of 3 phosphates. Vigorous exercise e.g. weights and sprinting, will soon use up ATP, after which Creatine Phosphate (CP) comes into play and it transfers its high energy phosphate to the Adenosine Phosphate (ADP), to restore what has been lost and endeavour to recreate ATP. CP, however, is also in short supply in muscles and the last source of energy will be glycogen - also consumed in an attempt to reproduce ATP. Glycogen is stored in the muscle in a long chain of glucose sugars. We are told each sugar molecule also has the energy to make 2 ATPs. Post the ATP - CP point, the Lactic-Acid System takes over. It should be noted, that tests have shown a marked decrease in CP and glycogen when training takes place in hot, humid conditions, so much so, that their replacement may take longer than 24 hours.

Like cars muscles, have fast and slow "motor units' which fire them into action and also different size 'motor units', basically the slower and smaller are used for non-maximum output and for longer periods. This division within muscle types has become to be known as the red **'Slow Twitch' (Type 1)** and the white **'Fast Twitch' (Type 2)** muscles. It's a bit of a broad generalisation as there would seem to be evidence for up to 7 types. FT develop tension rapidly, but cannot sustain it while ST develop tension slowly and are not easily fatigued. Basically, red, slow twitch fibers create what is known as aerobic activity, that is the extended effect of an endurance output - the principle energy source for this comes from fat. In contrast, white, fast twitch fibers perform anaerobic activity, or that of an explosive nature. It's only a very broad rule but any physical activity longer, in fact, than 10 seconds, can be regarded as endurance in nature, for which we use the red. Athletes who run, swim or cycle are practically all red. However, explosive sports ie. shotput, weights, short sprints, are where more white FT fibers will come into play.

Very broadly, slow twitch muscle cells are supplied with energy via oxygen in the blood. The fast cells use mainly the energy stored in the muscle (which is glucose). This is transformed into energy without oxygen and produces lactic acid as a by-product.

It's important to know that the type of muscle fibers one needs, determines the type of energy supply one needs. Each type of muscle fiber needs a particular energy source. The type of energy for this comes almost wholly from glycogen, which is derived from carbohydrate. As a runner, or endurance athlete, the energy source needs to come from things such as wheatgerm oil, vegetable oils, sunflower and safflower oils and also even fresh cream, as it is an easily digestible form of fat. In order to convert the fats, we need sufficient vitamins and particularly things like choline, inositol, Para Amino Benzoic Acid (PABA) and all 'B' complex vitamins.

Whether a fiber group is fast or slow depends upon its 'innervation' and its metabolic characteristics.

Note that it is not the 'speed' of movement, but requirement for heavy demand eg weight lifting, which brings the white fast twitch into play - slow movement plus POWER. Unfortunately, it would seem that a certain genetic unavoidability comes into the equation which we can do nothing about, in terms of being able to change the genetic make-up or fiber pattern, but what we can do is develop the metabolic potential of the various fibers.

In more aerobic types of training, muscles tend to grow longer and leaner, so more of the area is close to a supply route - tiny blood-carrying capillaries - at all times. Also, an aerobic conditioning programme, as described under the section about Blood, actually creates more supply routes.

To function muscles also need growth hormone, -- insulin, thyroid, testosterone and other hormones so as to develop naturally. Various hormones promote and stimulate amino acid transportation and protein synthesis and also, equally important, inhibit protein degradation. Adequate caloric and nutritive support is also necessary.

How does Exercise Stimulate Muscle Growth?
Well what we need to know is that exercise can operate alongside the normal endocrine system's effect in promoting muscle growth. Exercise effort can even influence muscle growth independently of calorific influence, ie irrespective of what

fuel we are taking in, in terms of food . As far as the skeletal muscles go and besides the proper nutritive and endocrine bases, chemical growth reactions favouring increased mass, are most heavily influenced by the 'intensity of effort'. How? - again the answer ends up containing words that look like a chemical formula, but the important factor in the process would seem to be Creatin which is both produced and utilised by muscular effort and which, in turn, stimulates the formulation of Myosin, a major muscle protein.

The traditional theory of muscle growth is that this occurs through what is known as hypertrophy, or increases in cross-section area without any additions of new muscle material. The theory goes on to state that the belief is that total fibre content is actually constant from birth. Another school of thought however does suggest the possibility that fibres can actually split (hyperplasia) and again by the process of hypertrophy there is an addition of connective tissue and what are referred to as 'satellite cell construction' towards new muscle tissues. However it happens, what we know is that correct exercise increases muscle size.

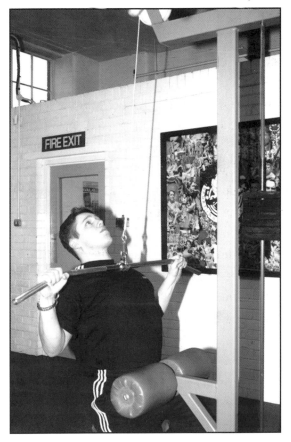

Wide grip lat pulldown – as with any weights exercise, you can design it to produce the results you want – vary weight, repetitions, or base your set on time!

Just finally on muscle growth, what must be remembered is that the above process is assisted through the deposition of proteins, increased water content and enhanced collagen deposits in and about the muscle fibres. Additionally, whilst myofibrillar proteins increase from exercise and cause hypertrophy, some research has revealed that the main increase in muscle weight comes from increased soluble or sarcoplasmic proteins (proteins separate from the actual contractile muscle fibres). Exercise increases the density of the actin and myosin proteins. Thus, exercise makes the muscles heavier, denser and not always bigger - but usually so.

The process is one by which muscle size is due to a combination of intricate damage and repair ie. over-compensation response (microtrauma, minute muscle tears, hydroxyproline build-up, lactic acid build-up, cell leakage, enhanced fluid content and a few others). This may come as a shock to some bodybuilders, but in support of some of the above, tests have shown bodybuilders have no more actual muscle fibres than untrained people.

How Fat Accumulates
All to do with metabolism and intake. Some people perform below par metabolically speaking, that is either too much food or a poor 'burn rate'. The obvious answer is to reduce the carbohydrate and fat intake or better utilise them. Studies show that most stored fat actually comes from under-utilised carbs.

Fats are actually easily assimilated and there are suggestions that on a fat and protein diet only, you won't actually get fat. Calories from carbs and calories from fats are different (see Chapter 4 - Nutrition). A good balance of all 3, together with a range of minerals and vitamins for the perfect utilisation of them. Any unused food intake is converted into Pyruvic Acid, which is the villain and which accumulates.

Fat is 'burned' by the 'Thermogenic' process of turning calories into heat. We actually accumulate different types of fat on our bodies, one being what is referred to as BAT (Brown Adipose Tissue). Supposedly BAT contains more blood vessels than normal fat and although it represents only 1% of total body tissue it produces as much heat (burned calories) as the rest of our body. BAT is high in mitochrondria - cellular energy producers - that burn fats and sugars. Supposedly it can burn its own weight in regular white fat in 12 hours.

Footnote: Products such as Lecithin are very good at helping fat utilisation and come in either powder, granules or capsule form.

Glycogen Resynthesis

Glycogen floods back into the muscles after hard exercise and also it comes back in greater concentration than had been in your muscles before the workout. We are told that this is highest during the first 2 hours after a workout and the best way to get the glycogen resynthesis happening, is to take in simple carbs - not complex. The main functionary in this is the liver and is the key organ in this resynthesis. The process is best served by the ingestion of fructose ie. sugars from fruit or in proprietary sports drinks.

Muscle Fatigue

Muscle fatigue will limit any performance, particularly endurance events. As with attempting to delay the lactic acid burn, the longer fatigue is delayed, the more you can do and perform. We should know how fatigue occurs so we can relook at diet and training to improve performance.

A good definition of muscle fatigue is *"**the failure of a muscle to maintain the required expected force/power output.**"*

There would seem to be 2 theories for fatigue. One is that the build-up of substances results in fatigue and two, that fatigue results from a depletion of substances and it is this one we look at first.

Depletion Theory

Evidence to support the depletion theory during anaerobic activity is not clear, however, it would seem to be well supported for aerobic work. As we know, during low intensity aerobic activity, slow twitch (slow oxidation) muscle fibres, are in the main, recruited. Glucose and free fatty acids (FFAs), which are stored in the muscle as glycogen and triglycerides, respectively, are the main fuel source.

Research would tend to suggest that stored body fat deposits are not depleted during low intensity exercise and will often last for days to fuel very long-term exercise. This somewhat contradicts the commonly held view, that after 20 minutes of aerobic exercise, we are 'burning' into fat reserves.

Muscle glycogen stores are, however, depleted with exercise. Once stored muscle glycogen is exhausted, blood glucose becomes an important fuel for aerobic exercise, but it can seldom maintain sufficient output by this means and fatigue occurs. The concept of stored muscle glycogen as a limiter to performance is supported by experiments involving low and high carb diets prior to exercise. A low carb intake has been shown to reduce endurance time, compared to that achieved after a normal diet. A high carb diet prior to exercise has been shown to increase muscle glycogen levels and to offset fatigue in long-term exercise - hence carbohydrate loading, which is now common among endurance athletes. The amount of glycogen stored by muscles can be increased by depleting stores and then replenishing them, causing overcompensation.

It should be remembered, however, that for every one carbohydrate molecule stored, two water molecules bind to it. The use of FFAs, possibly by ingestion of caffeine, helps reduce the calls on stored glycogen, as discussed earlier. The downside of caffeine, which is a diuretic, is that it may deplete fluid storage, which could cause problems during long endurance work in heat.

Moderate to high intensity exercise cannot be fuelled by FFAs but training can improve the body's choice of FFAs before glycogen, so sparing it. Training can also improve the ability of a muscle to use oxygen, enhance the local blood supply to the muscle and increase the efficiency of individual muscle cells.

Accumulation Theory

The accumulation of substances such as hydrogen ions (positively charged hydrogen atoms), ammonia and phosphates has also been shown to cause muscle fatigue. The build-up of hydrogen ions, particularly occurs in high-intensity, short duration, anaerobic exercise. As we now well know, fast twitch (fast glycotic) muscle fibers, are mainly used and 'anaerobic glycolysis' supplies energy during this type of exercise and results in the production of lactic acid, which is broken up into lactate and hydrogen ions. The demand, created by such intense effort, prohibits oxygen being used in the process as we learned earlier.

The accumulation of these causes muscle fatigue by slowing down important reactions in muscle cells, influencing the concentration of substances in the muscles, or, even influencing nerve pathways to the muscle. A build-up of ammonia has been shown to cause an overall increase in the lactic acid production and faster depletion of glycogen causing fatigue.

On a more theoretical front, there is a factor which has been called 'control fatigue' and this may result from the malfunction of nerve cells, where it is thought that a build-up of toxic substances during exercises may, in fact, cause decreased activity in areas of the brain responsible for initiating muscle activity. That having been said, a trainer's personal motivation and focus can have an important influence on muscle fatigue. The ability, through years of experience can enable a trainer to 'switch off', focus and push through the unpleasant feelings that muscle fatigue brings on. This does, in many ways, separate the good from the also-rans.

With many aspects of the 'human machine', our control, as exercised through our minds, is paramount in over-coming many of the unpleasant physical sensations which, ordinarily, may make us stop. This is commonly referred to as 'distress'.

We've all felt it at some time if we've put maximum effort into a physical effort, but we should still be capable of pushing the feeling down and not letting it affect us mentally. **The body will do what the body is designed to do - the mind will do what we have trained ourselves and it, to do.**

You should also know that with any exercise, the metabolisation of fat continues when exercise stops. In addition, your body will also make physiological changes in your metabolic rate (MR) increase.

Our resting metabolic rate (MBR) accounts for about 70% or more of our daily energy expenditure. The average person only burns between 100-150 calories every 10 minutes of exercise, whereas one piece of chocolate cake will contain some 400 calories. The benefit of exercise is that the MR remains a ccelerated after exercise, which can increase calorie burn by as much as 15%-50%. The more intense the exercise the more the increase and subsequent burn.

Our bodies should answer to our minds and our minds should answer to our willpower.

CHAPTER 4

NUTRITION

A good diet is 75% success in athletics and bodybuilding and, as such, it should be a major consideration for all of us who take training seriously.

A point to remember is that it's not what we eat, but what we can absorb that counts. A balanced diet means paying attention to all the items which make up the combination of nutrients - eg - **Proteins, Vitamins, Minerals, Enzymes, Fat, Trace Elements, Carbohydrates and absorbants**. People are different and sports are different. The subject matter of nutrition is difficult at times to understand and can be overly scientific. That having been said we should still endeavour to understand, as best we can, what it all means in simple terms and what we can do to achieve the best returns on what food we consume.

We talk about a balanced diet and essentially, this is about ensuring that the 3 main food groups, which we will look at below, are supplied in what can be called, an optimum amount. Lean protein, starchy (rice, potatoes, pasta) and fibrous (brocolli, green beans, spinach etc) carbohydrates and small amounts of fat and no sugar and little sodium.

Individual metabolism is a factor which makes any food balance a very personal thing, but as a broad guide, a heavy trainer's diet, where weights play a large part, would be 45 - 50% of calories from carbs, 35 - 40% from proteins and 10% - 15% from fat.

Also, a protein-rich diet, as we will see, raises the level of aminos, one consequence of which, is the production of neurotransmitters - dopamine and norepinephrine, which, so we are told, boost alertness, endurance and mental concentration.

The calorific benefit of the 3 major food groups are as follows:-

1 gramme of fat = 8/9 calories
1 gramme of protein = 4 calories
1 gramme of carbohydrate = 4 calories

Proteins. From the greek word meaning '**of primary importance**' proteins are the most important element, particularly for bodybuilders and strength athletes. The building blocks of the body, protein is usually required, by those who train, in larger amounts than that which would certainly be required for a sedentary person. Deterioration of muscle mass occurs when a deficiency is present.

We're told that a basic rule is 1 gram of 'first class' protein for 1 pound of body weight, plus 10% to cater for tissue replacement, broken down by hard muscular exercise. Made up of Amino acids which are chemically bonded together, proteins cannot enter the circulation and must be digested into their component parts - amino acids, or, very small chains of them.

There are 20 amino acids - 8 essential ie they cannot be manufactured by the body from other aminos. 1st class protein qualifies by dint of having all 8 amino acids, all the rest are not considered first class. Also some foods are better than others because of other factors - rated in biological value eg low water content, right amino acid balance and absorption. This includes -Eggs, Fish, Chicken, White meat, Red Meat. The most beneficial aminos are the 'L-aminos as they assist in the production of enzymes as well as hormone production.

At times an imbalance occurs, even in a balanced diet and we may feel the benefit of an amino-acid supplement. A mention should be made of Branched Chain Amino Acids (BCAA's). They have become popular as a supplement and differ from normal aminos in that they are metabolised in the muscle, whereas the others are broken down in the liver. Some 70% of the 'pool' of aminos utilised for repair is comprised of BCAA's. If training demands exceed energy supply aminos will be drawn from the muscle. Most supplementary aminos are 'pre-digested', in other words they don't need the same quantity of digestive enzymes such as pepsin.

Make your protein lean. Unfortunately, protein and fat usually co-exist in food. Diary produce and meat all have a counter-benefit. Move to low, non-fat sources eg. skimmed milk, egg whites, fish, chicken (no skin), or quality protein powders.

Of the above, eggs are best. They are the best assiminable, best combination of aminos, plus other substances such as Sulphur which assists in the absorption of protein as well as vitamin A, D and many of the B group. One Egg equals 6 grams of protein. We hear a lot about the problems of Cholesterol and most of it's bollocks. Cholesterol is a natural product (part of the Vitamain D group). If not consumed the body produces it. Cholesterol is a fat and the body needs fat to convert to energy, although like any fat it doesn't need too much of it. Cholesterol is no different, but in an active individual it is consumed from the bloodstream whereas in someone who enjoys an overly sedentary existence then excess over demand clogs up the arteries, narrowing them, which is not good. A cholesterol level of 300mg can be fatal and should be below 200mg.

Milk and goats milk, if we were to take 1 pint of it would contain about 12 grams of 1st class protein plus other elements, such as vitamins A, D, C and calcium and phosphate. Not everyone can, however, digest milk. Skimmed milk, for me, is one of the best foods. A good source of calcium, protein, vitamin D, and carbohydrate.

Fish - the highest protein in varieties comes from Tuna. Also the oil from fish is highly beneficial.

Chicken - high in protein, low in fat, no water, and easy to digest.

Red Meat - beef is high in protein but has a high water content. With protein, the best sources are usually the driest and, unfortunately, meat can be indigestible. NB. to help absorb protein, the body produces hydrochloric acid, pepsin and enzymes, which are normally produced in correct amounts, but with a high protein diet, sometimes additional aids are required. eg. Bromaline tablets - enzymes from pineapples.

Nitrogen Balance

As protein is eventually broken down into nitrogen, a positive balance means your body is absorbing it properly. To assist in maintaining a positive nitrogen balance, supplements such as alfalfa and kelp together, help the balance - kelp seems to stimulate the body. To assist in the body maintaining a correct nitrogen balance you must rest after a workout. It is also dangerous not to, as our vital organs are also depleted of necessary nitrogen

A positive nitrogen balance is the physiological state where muscle growth can take place. This can be achieved by small meals, taken regularly, eg every 2-3 hours, as distinct from 3 big ones.

Protein is digested and broken down into aminos and then into nitrogen and then used by the body for tissue repair and re-growth. Remember, the body needs to produce energy first, not strength or muscle growth. We need to ensure that the body has enough of the other basic nutritional requirements - carbohydrates and fat, from which it will have sufficient fuel for our body's energy requirements and, as a consequence, leave the protein alone. Many people who find muscular weight gain difficult, may not be getting sufficient carbohydrate.

Protein should be taken in small amounts during the day and we are told that the human body can only absorb approx, 30 grams at one sitting, so small amounts a day assure better assimilation.

When we eat, our metabolic rate increases, as chemical processes concerned with digestion occur. However, the chemical processes which deal with the amino acids require even more energy and increase the MR to an even greater extent. By comparison, taking in protein raises the metabolic rate by as much as 30%, for as long as 12 hours - whereas carbohydrates will move the MR up by only 4%. To enhance this effect, eat protein in small quantities, regularly during the day.

Protein is also loaded with the amino acid Tyrosine, which helps make the brains neurotransmitter Noreprinephine (like adrenaline), which is crucial to quick thinking, fast reactions and a feeling of good concentration and alertness. Proteins provide a good mental energy.

Carbohydrates

For the most part all the Carbohydrates are made from 3 single sugars (Monosaccharides) - Glocuse, Fructose and Glucose. These are the only sugars which can enter your circulation and be used for calories - also they must be digested before use. Ordinary sugar (sucrose) is digested into glucose and fructose. The carbs, in milk, for example, are digested into gluctose and gulactose. The starches and glycogen are larger molecules composed entirely of glucose whilst Cellulose ie the walls of plants cannot be digested by the human body and provides bulk, but no energy. The sugars in pure honey is actually pre-digested sucrose and is present as the single sugars glucose and fructose.

Average daily consumption should never be below 100gms or 800 calories and for hard training 500 - 700 gms, that is some 2,000 - 2,800 calories. Carbohydrates are energy foods. They are broken down by the B vitamins and converted to energy. Carbohydrates can be obtained from a variety of sources such as fruit, vegetables, rice, etc etc.

Carbohydrates are essential to properly digest protein. When carbs are eaten, the body converts it to glucose, which in turn then convert aminos into nitrogen, which is the end product of protein. If there are no carbs present in a diet, then the liner converts the amino acid, not into nitrogen but into glucose to act as an energy fuel and then into urea, which is excreted from the body, but there is no tissue growth.

When we train, muscles burn oxygen. Oxygen is contained in the body's red blood corpuscles and the more red blood cells you have, the more oxygen transport you have. 70% of red blood cells are composed of haemoglobin and Iron is vital to all living cells because of its function of transporting oxygen. Another 70% feature is that this is the amount which the body stores its Iron in the muscles - the rest being stored in the liver. A diet high in fat and sugar can actually deplete a body's natural store of Iron. Later, we will look at building reserves for high intensity workouts.

Medium Chain Triglycerides (MCTs)

These are a form of fat, which take on the attributes of carbs, which is achieved by removing a number of carbon atoms. This allows the body to use the reformed substance as an energy source and prevents storage as fat. It's a good supplement for bodybuilders. We know that carbohydrates are converted into glycogen, which is the preferred energy source, particularly for bodybuilding, but intense training, will deplete these glycogen stores and the body then unfortunately, can burn muscle tissue for energy. Using MCTs can offset this and are useful also as a weight gainer.

Pre-Workout Lactic Acid Buffer

During intense workouts, we are all familiar with the burning sensation we feel in our muscles, especially with high reps. This is not a muscle ache, but lactic acid burn. As a consequence, many a set is stopped before the muscle is totally worked, due to the pain of the burn. Lactic acid build-up is inevitable, but can be postponed. Such elements as Bicarbonate, Phosphate and Carnosine will help reduce the burn, allowing more work.

Muscle contraction is the province of ATP - this is the fuel which helps a muscle contract. With high output, there can be a combination of both lactic acid burn and oxygen debt eg. breathlessness. Lactic acid build-up, apart from the pain, has other drawbacks. High acidity in the blood, detracts from the ability of cells to produce ATP, needed for muscle contractions. Since there is no way to prevent it forming, the best solution is to delay it's onset. Even small doses of bicarbonate of soda delays its onset and presents a 'buffering' effect in the blood, while Phosphate and

Carnosine have a 'buffering' effect in the muscle itself. Combined together in capsule form for pre-workout, they come highly recommended.

Carbohydrate loading should take place 24 hours before a heavy endurance event eg. marathon or fell run, to ensure maximum reserves of glycogen in the muscles.

The downside of carbohydrates is in fact a 'mental' downside - by this, I mean that a carbohydrate intake, whilst providing eventually the glycogen stores, can, in the short term, leave us less than mentally stimulated and often lacking the desire to train. The reason is that carbs produce Tryptophan, an amino acid which is used in the brain to make the neurotransmitter - serotonin, a chemical messenger that reduces our ability to concentrate, slows reaction time and makes us sleepy.

On the plus side, unlike fat, if we end up with a 200 calorie excess of carbs from our diet, a full 60 calories would be used up in the conversion of the excess carbs to stored body fat - some 30% are used up in the process. Avoid simple carbs from sugar or any sucrose-laden food. This causes a dramatic rise in blood sugar levels, which in turn, creates an over-abundance of insulin. The result is the insulin takes too much sugar out of our bloodstream, causing us to feel tired, weak, irritable and also hungry again. Complex carbs, pasta, potatoes and rice, for example, are broken down slowly in our digestive system, creating a more steady release of insulin. Also, too much simple sugars can cause fat retention, due again to excess insulin.

Post Training
We should ingest carbs and protein shortly after training to maximise muscle growth and replace spent energy stores. Supposedly, we need both immediately after training and again, at a point some 2 hours later.

Insulin and cortisol, the 2 most potent of the body's anabolic and catabolic hormones respectively, need to be unbalanced in favour of the anabolic effect of insulin (within reason), to produce the body's correct nitrogen balance. Exercise increases the body's efficiency in metabolising carbs, but often intense exercise causes the 'stress hormones' to break down aminos as a secondary energy source.

Carbohydrates alone, taken after training, are not sufficient in their own right to promote adequate increases in glycogen storage. Protein is now thought to be essential, combined with carbs to achieve the best result. Care is needed, however, not to overlook the need to continue with the intake for some hours later, as the increased carb uptake, due to the protein, can cause a very large drop in 'blood sugar' or 'hypoglycaemia'.

Fats

Fats, these days, are variously categorised as mono-unsaturated, poly-unsaturated and saturated. Saturated fats, which cause a build-up of blood cholesterol and which are implicated in hypertension, heart disease and strokes, should be avoided. We need fats in our diet for absorption of fat soluble vitamins ie. A, D, E and K and we also need fat for energy, but we don't need saturated fats for these processes.

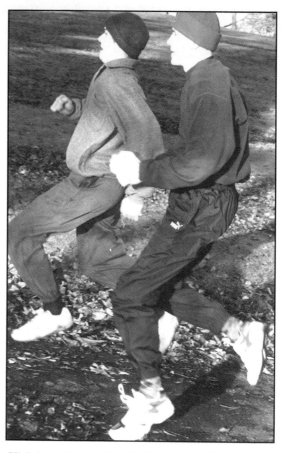

High knee lifts, combined with the other hill work, will cause glycogen starvation. Ensure you are replacing losses through nutrition - prior, during and after.

Dietary fat is more easily converted and stored as body fat, but remember, excess protein and also carbs, will eventually be converted into fat stores. Dietary fat though, needs no other process, nor does it use up much energy to change into body fat. Dietary fat is very simply made into a triglyceride and moved into your fat cells. 200 calories of extra fat, will probably store as 200 calories of body fat.

Remember, fat is only oxidised through aerobic effort - in other words, only endurance-type exercise, over reasonably long periods will eventually 'burn fat'.

Don't, however, be afraid of a sensible consumption of fats which are referred to as **'High Density Lipoproteins' (HDLs),** as these help carry away the dangerous **'Low Density Lipoproteins'** - cholesterol from our arteries. Be careful when viewing consumption of meat or other products, particularly when taking fat content as a percentage of weight. A product which has 3% fat by weight may still have 30% fat by calories. Don't be fooled with supposed low fat products. On the positive side, fish oils have a very beneficial effect, not least, we are now told, in fighting cancer and help reducing the risk of cardio-vascular diseases. In addition, fish oils also have a beneficial effect on joints. Omega 3, the fatty acids from fish oil, are the good fats here.

A current school of scientific thought is that it isn't actually fat which makes you 'fat', but excess insulin released by eating too many carbs in one sitting, or too many calories in one meal. Whilst we all need insulin release to enable us to get sugars and aminos into our cells, a bi-product is the inhibition of fat mobilisation and oxidation - in other words, the body's ability to burn and use fat.

It helps, if we ensure our fat intake is linked to the mono-unsaturated type, which are themselves based on HDL or 'good cholesterol'. HDLs are thought to prevent both cardio-vascular disease and cancer. Olives, Olive Oil, Nuts, Avocados are all sources of mono-unsaturates.

Read the labels more on the food you eat. Also remember when you're reading the constituent nature of fat in a product, that one gramme of fat is still one gramme of fat, irrespective of whether its a 'good fat' or a 'bad saturated fat'.

We are told the average male carries about 100,000 calories of stored fat, as distinct from approx. 1,600-2,000 as carbohydrates. Tests with U.S. army rangers showed that too low a % body fat was unhealthy and lead to poor physical and mental performance. The conclusion was that 4 - 6% body fat *"represents the lower limit for healthy men"*. This, is in contrast to some bodybuilders who foolishly endeavour to get below this.

Fats are a combination of fatty acids and glycerol and most fat is stored as neutral fat, or triglycerides - 3 fatty acids are attached to one glycerol molecule. Fats cannot be absorbed either, unless digested, breaking down the fat molecule into fatty acids. You should know that food that contains lots of fats are not a good source of immediate energy because the energy is not available until digestion has taken place and complete. Fats are the slowest of all food components to be digested and absorbed. Fat is digested by 'pancreatic lipase'. This enzyme breaks down 'neutral' fat - mostly triglycerides into single fatty acids. This is why you can't ingest special fats such as lecithin - it must be digested into component fatty acids and glycerol parts.

Just touching for a moment on vitamins and their relationship with fat, vitamins D, E and K depend on the absorption of fat to enter the internal body, but only relatively small amounts are required for this purpose.

Vitamins
Proteins are the building blocks and vitamins are the glue or cement, which binds them together.

Vit A - Easiest to obtain in a good diet. Essential for skin, eyes, and needed to fully utilise protein. Vegetables, milk, eggs, liver and in fish - liver oils, ie. halibut and cod.
Vit B - This is a complex or family of vitamins and probably the most important for an athlete. Vitamin B has many tasks as it creates enzymes in the body for the full utilisation of carbs, starch, fat and protein. Obtainable from dessicated liver, brewers yeast, wholewheat, wheatgerm.
Vit C - The muscle cement vitamin. It has a tightening effect on the muscle tissue, due to the excretion of excess water, as C is a natural diuretic. Cleanses and helps against stress, plus it creates adrenal hormones for strength and endurance. It is not stored so would be required every day. We need in excess of 1,000mg per day, to be effective.

Vit D - Needed to facilitate the absorption of calcium and other minerals eg. from fish and liver oils, but also in eggs and milk. Sunshine activates the formation of Vitamin D in the body.

Vit E - The 'Youth' vitamin, supposedly it increases virility and also increases endurance. We are told that E allows the muscles to work with less oxygen. Found in wheatgerm oil, wholewheat. Vitamin B12 - anti-anaemic - helps produce red blood cells.

The above is only representative and not a comprehensive list of all vitamins or sources.

Minerals

Minerals are like vitamins, they aid the body in the absorption and utilisation of the food we consume.

Calcium - bones, teeth, nerves and blood. From milk, cheese, butter and most dairy produce.

Phosphate - acts with calcium. From meat.

Magnesium - helps reduce cholesterol, plus a high intake for athletes seems to produce strength gains. Mostly in green vegetables, some in milk and dairy produce.

Potassium - feeds the muscles and benefits the blood. From fresh fruit - oranges etc.

Iron - creates red blood corpuscles and helps the absorption of protein. From liver and eggs etc.

Copper - works with iron. See Iron.

Iodine - regulates the thyroid gland and acts with starch and carbohydrates. From seafood, particularly shell fish and kelp.

Zinc - the body needs 2 x as much zinc as it does Iron. It seems to be a great repairer of muscle tissue and is used in hospitals. From honey.

Chelation - for minerals to be absorbed, they need to go through a process called 'chelation'. This means that the minerals are surrounded by aminos, broken down and absorbed. Although this naturally takes place in the body, it is now possible to get mineral supplements in this form.

Fruit

Fruit is an essential in a balanced diet and provides magnesium, potassium, chromium and many other nutrients eg.

    Bananas - a medium banana has 0.3gm of fibre, Vit B6 and potassium.
    Apples - 1 large apple has 4.0gm of fibre.
    Pineapples - 0.8gms of fibre, potassium, Vit A, and is invaluable in the
                    digestive process of protein.
    Oranges - potassium and Vit C.

Vegetables

    Spinach, Brocolli, Carrots and Tomatoes, between them contain Vitamin C, A,
    B6, Magnesium, Potassium, Calcium and Fibre.
    Potatoes - Vit B6, C and Iron, as well as the obvious carbohydrate value.

Energy For Anaerobic Activity

In Chapter 3 - 'The Human Machine', we looked in some detail at the functioning of the body and what nutrients were required, particularly those that fuelled activity. We looked at the use of fats for long-term endurance events, but when requiring to be fit to fight, our principle activity will usually be somewhat more anaerobic and, as a consequence, we will be in a state of oxygen debt.

Our primary energy source when we have 'gone' anaerobic, is glycogen, which is really a form of natural sugar. The body can store glycogen, so if you have a high body store, you can train with good intensity. Our primary food source for this are the 'complex' carbohydrates, not carbs from sources such as sugar or white flour products. Better sources would be wholewheat bread, rice, pasta, wholegrain cereals, dates, figs, apples, bananas, together wih a good selection of vitamins, which are invaluable for perfect utilisation of carbs.

NB. Levulose, a natural fruit sugar is a very good source of energy. The great advantage of this product is the fact that it bypasses the normal digestive programme associated with other ordinary sugar. Other forms of sugar ie. sucrose, dextrose, glucose and the like, all require insulin in order to digest them, so that the body can either use them as an energy source or exude them. Levulose and fructose don't need insulin, so they pass quickly into the bloodstream, providing an immediate energy source, but also in a steady, controlled manner.

It's important to avoid food supplements described as energy products, which contain glucose and sucrose, as they will eventually, through the complex process of insulin production, actually lower the blood sugar level.

Any excess food element, whether it is from starch, carbohydrate, fat or protein, is stored in the body's tissues if not used up - in other words - stored as bodyfat.

The body will guard glycogen in the muscles and will use other sources of energy in place. Fat will be one of the primary sources of energy and a normal uptake would be some 20%, however, the presence of caffeine can boost this up to 40%, the consequence of which is to extend endurance, as you will make glycogen last longer and also burn more fat. The suggestion is, therefore, to drink a cup of coffee one hour before you train.

Water in Sports

Basically, you need more than you are probably getting. The most important nutrient of all that we can take in. It's a misconception that a high water intake makes us bloated - just the opposite. Our body's defence mechanism makes us 'hold water' when our intake falls. Keep your water intake up - that's water not fluid intake.

Energy For Muscle Building

As we know, muscles are built by resistance exercise such as weight training. Tissue is broken down and replaced by nature, which also adds a bit so as to compensate. Nutritionally, the process is like this. The insulin in the system directs amino acids into the muscles, stimulating cell growth. The technical term is called 'enlarging of the myofibrils' and as mentioned above, insulin is also associated with blood sugar levels.

Glycogen within the muscles actually raises blood sugar, or in effect promotes the creation of insulin, which in turn motivates the aminos into the muscle tissue eg.

- **complex carbs build up glycogen**
- **glycogen raises blood sugar levels and promotes insulin**
- **insulin drives aminos into the muscles**
- **the muscle responds by enlarging**

A side effect of training is a lowered blood sugar level, which acts to deplete the body's store of insulin. Glycogen is extracted from the muscles in order to try and restore the insulin level, so it can continue to supply the muscle with aminos, however, as training continues, the supply of glycogen is also depleted. Insulin production stops or slows and the muscle stops receiving aminos.

The key factor therefore, is to keep blood sugar levels as high as possible for as long as you can. To that end, we need to have supplied our body with complex carbohydrates and, between training sessions, we must ensure a regular supply of carbs to allow our body to continue to store glycogen. After training for about 3/4 hour, our blood sugar level drops to a figure of 90, whereas to successfully create muscle growth, it should be maintained at a level of 140. Any assistance from honey, fructose tablets, levulose or a range of training drinks, will help. If you have supplied your body consistently with complex carbohydrates and the sessions don't exceed one hour, you should be okay. Wheat and brewers yeast help regulate insulin levels in the system.

Lean body mass, activity levels, hormone levels and the genetics we inherit, all have a part to play in the rate of metabolism. As mentioned above, insulin levels can play a major role in fat storage and this is where the **glycemic index** comes into play.

For a moment it is worth looking in more detail at insulin, which is essentially a protein hormone. It is released by the beta cells of the pancreas in response to sugar and aminos in the bloodstream. Much of its importance is that it facilitates transport of carbohydrates and aminos into the muscle. This, as we illustrated above, promotes the synthesis of muscle glycogen. The problem with insulin however, is that while it promotes growth, it promotes fat storage. Insulin release, stimulates the enzyme Lipoprotein Lipase, which plays a key role in fat synthesis and insulin can also inhibit other fat burning enzymes.

It is worth remembering that big meals are supposed to cause an 'insulin rush' and we are told that it is better, as a consequence, to eat 6 smaller meals than 3 big ones, which both lowers insulin levels and regulates the release of blood sugar into the blood.

The glycemic index, which we mentioned above, was developed to help diabetics. Essentially, it measures how rapidly carbohydrates are digested and stored. The faster a carb breaks down, the more insulin is released and the easier fat is deposited NB. the higher the number, the more insulin released, the lower = less. Those people whose goal is to have lean mass, yet grow, need to ingest those carbs with 50 or less. Rice Cakes, of all things, with a number 133 on the index is like pure sugar. Pasta at 60 on the index is far better than rice at 82. Potatoes with an index of 80 is also at the upper end of the scale.

That having been said, some people have a regular insulin release, however and whatever they eat, whereas others may experience a subsequent drop in blood sugar, leaving them listless and exhausted. To help things in your favour, if you reduce your body fat, your system will secrete less insulin for any given amount of carbs. Also, an intake of fibre retards the breakdown of carbs, by slowing glucose entry into the bloodstream. Also, it seems to be understood that higher blood sugar levels suppress growth hormone. In adults, the biggest release of growth hormone is during the first 90 minutes of sleep and to maximise the effect, limit your carb intake for at least 3 hours before retiring and make them carbs at the low end of the scale.

Supplements
Even in a balanced diet, often there are some cracks, down which our perfect and complete nutritious intake of essential elements falls. Supplements are a way of

filling in those cracks. Often the problem is not knowing what we are short of, or missing out in our diet and this book cannot confess to be the place to look in any detail at the efficacy of vitamin, mineral, or other supplements. On a personal front, I take cod liver oil, vitamin C, although not with the regularity I know I should. Over the years and in short bursts, I've taken brewers yeast, dessicated liver and a range of other supplements, without, I have to say, any noticeable effect.

What we must remember, however, is how a body fuels its workouts. By using supplements before a workout such as **pre-digested liquid meals (PDLM's),** we can raise the bodies insulin level, which, as an anabolic hormone increases the uptake of amino acids and glucose which will assist in the muscles growth. A bi-product is that by doing this we also 'spare' the muscle protein from breaking down during the workout. PDLM's can come in liquid form or as powder to mix with water, milk or fruit juices. They are made from major energy sources such as protein, carbohydrate and fat and are pre-digested to varying degrees by the use of enzymes or acids to break them down and make them more easily digestible. This process breaks down major nutrients into smaller molecular units.

The form the PDLM's take is in aminos from **protein**, MCT's (medium-chain triglycerides) or, as it is known, 'fatless fat' from **fat** and usually Glucose polymers from **carbohydrate** sources such as corn starch. The latter is far more effective in replacing depleted glycogen stores than simple sugar products.

After workouts, supplements can help 'jump start' the recovery process, by initiating glycogen and muscle protein synthesis. Endurance training, particularly, tends to break down muscle. We understand, that studies show some 5-10% of the body's energy needs during aerobic exercise are met through amino acid oxidation, in other words, being burnt for energy. This, we are told, is because the body inter-prets intensive aerobic work as akin to starvation, which promotes the breakdown of muscle for energy. This process can be halted by ensuring we have sufficient levels of liver glycogen stores to assist in maintaining the anabolic hormones.

Supplements such as amino acid mixtures, carbohydrate drinks and powders, protein powders, MCT and metabolic optimisers, weight gain powder etc all help in loading insulin, maintaining the nitrogen balance and spare protein. If we are sweating a lot during exercise I feel it is essential that we take some sort of carbo-electrolyte drink. Such solutions are better absorbed than just water alone to counter the effects of dehydration and the electrolytes are absorbed, we are told, some six times faster if carbohydrates are present.

Whether we are taking magnesium, lost through sweating, or extra vitamin E, to safeguard the oxygen supply to the muscles, in some way we do benefit our bodies in their complex biology and functioning. Whilst I'm sure on many occasions, the benefit is psychosomatic and the clinical gains negligible or nil, but what the hell - I think they work.

CHAPTER 5

RUNNING

I started running in a serious way to increase my fitness at about nineteen'ish!. At that time I was a member of the Gt. Britain and England Karate squads and up till then I'd had four years of traditional Karate and what fitness I'd derived had been solely from that. I used a public park near where I lived in Manchester and made use of an outdoor cinder running track - in fact I did more 'shuttles' across one of the wide bends than I did laps around it. I still didn't put many miles in and even then I think I realised my requirement for a certain type of fitness, although at that juncture could not define it in the very specific terms I know it now.

If I seem in this chapter to be taking a somewhat askance view of running then you may have missed the point, as running has been one of the mainstays in my training programme. Wherever I've been in the world I've tried to create a circuit. You will, however, be left in no doubt, that if I felt I didn't have to run, I probably wouldn't do it.

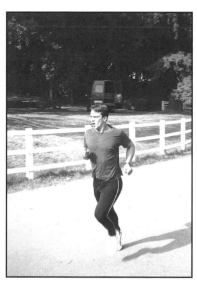

Running is probably the basis of all aerobic activity we do. Here - a good, light step.

It doesn't matter where you are or what else you can't do you can usually always run. I've run when I've been working in such diverse places as Moscow, Kiev, Beirut, Kazakhstan, Algeria and all points East and West. I've run in snow, ice, fog driving wind and rain and desert conditions and like all other training, the harsher the environment the more the 'hardening' process is at work. I'm often happier running in the rain as I can cut out my surroundings and run in my own cocoon.

What Is Running?

We talk of jogging, sprinting, long-slow-distance, pacing and fartlek and a whole host of other variations to the basic theme of putting one foot in front of the other at a faster pace than we do if we had to walk somewhere. In a way that's the beauty of running - it can be all things to all people.

It can be a fat burner, or a way of gaining size. It can improve basic cardio-vascular capacity or anaerobic capability and it can take place on the flat, on hills, on tarmac, on grass, sand, fellside or indoors and on machines. But probably above all attributes the greatest one which running has is that its free. You pay no one to do it and with the minimum amount of kit - which can last for years (decades in my case), it's probably the cheapest way to stay fit that I know.

I've always found running hard, but I've benefited over the years by training with people who were not half bad runners. Running is something we all think we can do quite naturally without having to consider technique or purpose, other than to move one foot in front of the other at a faster pace than we walk and, magically, get fit. In the good old days I never carried excess body weight and any volume of distance work would have been detrimental to the maintenance of size. Also, and this is where running gets difficult for me, my boredom threshold is very low, particularly when running - half an hour and that's it! On a flat course for me that's about four and a half miles and, with some moderate to steepish inclines on the route, will extend to some 35/40 minutes. That's my ideal run, at the end of which I'm losing it mentally.

If that run precedes a full workout afterwards then it's more than enough. For many years my Sunday morning sessions were 35 minutes of a hilly circuit, in a park in Manchester, literally a walk across the road into my training partner's garage, then bagwork, pad work and sparring. The whole session was 2 hours religiously. The effort needed was high and it was a taxing session. We conducted the run competitively and even when it didn't start off that way, it would usually end like that. It was a hilly circuit and took a good level of mental resolve to push through to the end.

Remember - once you're over 20 minutes of exercise and it's within your aerobic threshold, then you're burning fat. For me, this is one of the primary benefits. Running over average distances is one of my mainstays for keeping bodyfat down and the cardiovascular system working at peak capacity. I've put in big distances and taken part in 2 **Karrimor** and 1 **Saunders Mountain Marathon** in the '80's, after a couple of years of intense hill-walking with weight. These events comprise 2-man teams running (and walking) over 2 days in mountainous and difficult terrain, carrying enough to survive on. This includes a tent, sleeping bags, food etc and navigation plays as much a part as fell-running ability and fitness. These are a variation of the long 'O' or long orienteering events, it's just that the race is a team one over 2 days. It has to be one of the hardest sporting events without going 'extreme' and even to finish is an accomplishment. Orienteering itself is also one of the most demanding of sports with ever changing pace and terrain to fight through. The attraction of the hills is never lost to me and if I have a choice I'll drive some way to a suitable rural training ground rather than pound the city streets.

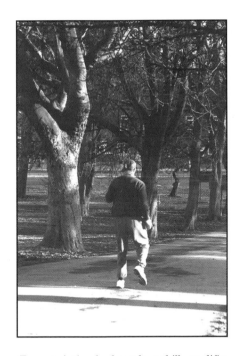

Even sprinting backwards, uphill, qualifies as running.

Training for such an event as the Karrimor is time-consuming and all-consuming. You have to 'train specific' - in other words, 4 miles around the streets, 3/4 times a week won't do any good at all. If you want to survive a long distance fell run, you've got to run on the fells. This means time and dedication. It leaves no time for other training, without becoming a complete social outcast. However, as a test of one's mental and physical endurance and the strength of friendship - there's nothing quite like it - even when I was caught up in it I did everything else.

Environment

The running routine I've had for many years has always evolved from the environment and locations I've had to train in. For many years I've been able to find locations which held everything, particularly undulating and hilly terrain, either road or off-road, that can be taken in a circuit and with which one can also adapt the terrain for hill-sprints or hill-carry work. I don't combine a 4.5 miler with hill-sprints if I can help it, unless its a flat 4.5 miles. If it's an up and down course and if it's taxing I won't sprint, although I'll always follow it with a secondary training session.

When I'm hill-sprinting or doing work on steps, then I only want half to three-quarters of a mile outrun to the hill just to warm up and loosen things and it's jogged at a moderate rate. Also I know full-well that when I'm finished I'm only just able to walk, let along run 2 to 3 miles back to the car. Park that half to 1 mile away and then you've got a natural warm-up and cool-down after the anaerobic work.

If all you've got for distance work is a flat course, then 'up the pace'. Bring the time down and get a good stride pattern going. Always start easy - get your breathing into a groove and your back and legs stretched and relaxed. The first mile should be at an average pace, then open up for at least a mile and a half and then ease back for half a mile and then hit the last section. Get a good long stride pattern and eat the distance. Get the feeling you're flying and whilst it's a personal thing for me, running on the balls of the feet without the heel ever touching, always gives me the lightest feeling. This last section should make up, time-wise, for the first mile which is kept down in pace. You should know you've got a fast finish in you and again, hit it for the last 100 metres. At times you'll be reaching your aerobic threshold, but don't worry because each time you're out pushing it, you're extending the barrier at which you will go anaerobic.

All Things To All People

The beauty of running is that it can serve a number of purposes. If you want to satisfy a desire for fitness without distress, you can go for 'long slow distance' work. If you want to 'add on' to a heavy strength regime, you can use it to burn fat or can structure your running to be a mainstay of your power - strength - explosive development. Compare the physique of a 100 and 200 metre runner with that of a 3,000, 10,000 or marathon runner and think which you'd probably rather have if you had to get into a fight. You probably know from experience that a fight isn't going to last for 2.5 hours or for 10 minutes - it'll probably be over in 10 to 30 seconds if someone's halfway competent, but in that short space of time the effort it may take could be completely exhausting and not dissimilar from that 100 metre sprint. It will stress the musculature to the point of being almost non-functional and it will place demands on the cardiovascular system that often can't be met, particularly with the fear, stress, indecision, adrenalin and minor symptoms of shock. Once the fight starts you feel as if you're at the 300 metre point of a 400 metre sprint - in other words - exhausted.

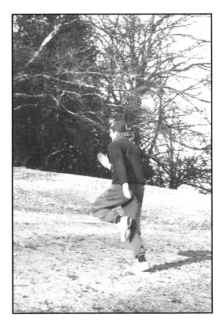

We're told that the 400 metre race is one where, for the first 300 metres it's possible for the runners to be performing aerobically, however, for the last 100 metres they've gone anaerobic and run on pure willpower, aggression, determination and the physical ability to operate within the

The last few metres of a 150 metre hill sprint - now it's mental.

anaerobic threshold. YOUR FIGHT STARTS AT THAT 300 METRE POINT. You can't ease into a fight in the street - it's explosive, urgent, terrifying and violent. It may involve grapplng, striking - pushing and pulling and anything that comes to the forefront of your mind as a trained response. The one who wins is not the one who is a better technician, but the one who is not prepared, under that dread feeling of emptiness and despair, to stop and give in.

A fight is like one of those international sprints where hundredths of seconds separate the places. In a fight, one man is a tenth or a hundredth of second away from giving up. Unfortunately, the opponent has no way of knowing that's all that separates them or how close his opponent is from giving up and sadly he may, without that knowledge give up first - literally the fight as we say, goes out of him. So remember if you give up it was probably a fraction of a second before your opponent would have. It's all too easy to believe that in a fight or a confrontation, you're the only one who's frightened, distressed or run out of breath. The skill is in not showing it.

"A MAN IS NOT FINISHED WHEN HE'S DEFEATED - HE'S FINISHED WHEN HE LEAVES THE ARENA". (A quote from the film - 'Lillehammer Winter Olympics 1994')

The purpose of hill-work and sprint-training is to create a feeling of distress which equates with that you will feel during a real conflict. What you're trying to achieve is a familiarity with distress and then to be able to function and perform physically even when your body can't - **IT IS YOUR MIND THAT CONTROLS EVERYTHING - NOT YOUR BODY.**

Whilst on the subject of 400metre running, we couldn't pass by without a look at Michael Johnson - now 200 and 400metre Olympic champion. His style and technique seems to defy all the traditional thinking that used to prevail in sprinting. With his college coach, Clyde Hart, they found that his very erect posture seemed to conserve energy and his 'on the toes' running style, with a consequent low knee lift, all seem to contribute to a very deceptively fast pace. Maybe all this conservation of effort is what delays the onset of 'blood lactate' accumulation, which is building up between the 300+ mark and the finish. The lactate acid, as we know, inhibits the free passage of nerve impulses to the muscle fibres and, as a consequence, the rate at which muscles contract. 'Tying up', on the home straight, is literally what happens and the paradox is that the harder at that point an athlete tries, the more he contributes to a slower pace still.

Johnson's strategy is to get the first 200metres in as comfortable and rhythmic a pace as possible. Interestingly, when training, he also never runs flat out sprints, but strives for strength and endurance.

By training past the aerobic threshold, you're duplicating combat conditions and pro-gramming your mind so that it is familiar territory for it and that you know deep down if you are in a conflict and feel like giving up, you still have something left. Even on empty, your tank will be fuelled with memory. This is how 400m runners manage that last 100m and how you should approach a fight. Your

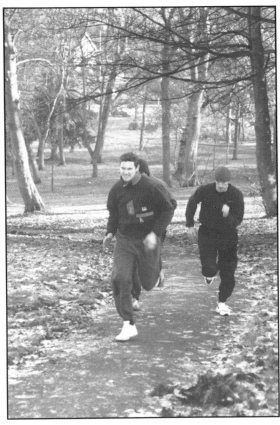

Now it's competitive! and you had better have some good sprinting technique - keep relaxed and focus only on yourself and your technique - ignore everyone else.

first '300 metres of a fight', goes very quickly with the onset of fear and the adrenal rush and all the other attendant factors. Once you start to fight, you can quickly move into that anaerobic zone where you think it's all over for you.

Providing you don't show distress you can still win. Your opponent will be just as bad, if not worse, and he'll probably show how bad it is for him with facial expressions, therefore when you train, use the opportunity to ensure you don't show distress. After your sprint don't squat down, fall to your knees or give the game away with a pained expression on your face. Your training is as much about personal control as it is about physical exertion. When you finish a hill-sprint or hill-carry, resist the temptation to sit, squat or lean forward with your hands on your knees - stand, put your hands on your hips and try and get the air in that you need, in a steady manner. Even if you're not, look as if you're ready to go again - use this as a training session in how you will eventually psyche someone out.

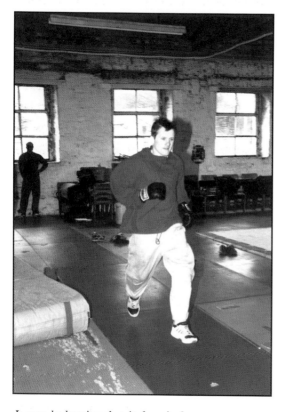

It may be hurting, but it doesn't show.

Many fights are over and lost as a result of one person simply having a better presentation than the other person. What I mean by presentation is the overall image conveyed - bearing, aggression, facial expression, vocal use etc. All these form part of the process of mental domination, even if that domination at the time feels as if its based on a foundation of sand. I've known many skillful combatants, who were physically and technically fairly poor, but they made up for it in their presentation skills. Opponents believed that they must be world-beating if their attitude was anything to go by. Many conflicts can be resolved by a confident attitude, linked with good verbal skills (see *'Streetwise'* by the author).

Focus

Like all training where you exceed your aerobic capacity and your muscles are starting to seize up, only controlled aggression and focus will see you through. If you are hill-sprinting or hill-carrying you can see the top of the hill - it may only be another 10 paces, but often even at that short distance it's still possible to quit and this is because the focus has been lost. Focus is the concentration you must give to the task in hand to the exclusion of all other thoughts. What happens normally is that as you start to get distressed, negative emotions start to set in. As you sprint for the top of the hill, you may be passed by someone or you may be unable to catch someone if you're in a 'hare and hounds' practice.

Negative emotions start to happen sub-consciously, not consciously, and we begin to slow down or stop. If it's at that point where the legs are wobbling or your heart's about to burst - or so you think - then the negative emotions set in and our mind dwells on whether we will be able to do the next set of exercises and tries to modify the output during the one we're currently in. At this point, how focused you are will determine whether you quit or push through.

When training, it always seems innocent enough to allow these verbal messages about balancing effort to have some place, but it's not, because it sets up a mental programming which is both insidious and malignant, because what will happen is that when it comes to that fight, you'll quit because your sub-conscious is pro-grammed, through your training, to simply quit at the 8/10ths or 9/10ths mark too often before.

So what you have to guard against is not setting training regimes and drills that are simply too ambitious, too soon. Having said that, don't use that statement as an excuse for not making your sessions hard as well as physically and mentally taxing, it's simply about getting the correct balance. Don't think from all this that everytime I go out I never fail - I do, for a variety of reasons, but if I do I know that the session was a hard one so I've not mislead nor deceived myself. Also, whilst I may not make it all the time, I'll never be accused of not setting hard training goals. What I do know well enough about myself is that failure at an exercise strengthens my resolve, not the reverse. I come back the next time, determined not to fail and remember this, you will always have good and bad days. Some days, unaccountably, performance is less than good. This may be due to mental, physical, diet, or any number of issues in combination but whatever, you need to know you have at least put in 120% each time.

Always be ready to train, particularly if you train with others. If you've committed yourself to train with someone else, then however you feel, you ensure that a negative attitude doesn't infect others. The balance between success and failure in a hard training session for people is very fine and a negative and non-committed attitude by someone is destructive for everyone. When you train - SHOW SPIRIT. You do this by your aggressive approach and by your general positive attitude.

Running has never come easy to me. As I've said earlier, I have a low boredom threshold and running any distance requires normally the accompaniment of a Walkman and motivational music. With any distance work I need the buzz from music, but what I do find is that I can't sprint or hill-climb any distance listening to a Walkman. For some reason the music beat and the increased hard breathing rate seem to fight each other and my breathing loses out. This is only when sprinting, but it seems to affect me, so be aware if you run to music.

This book does not aim to dwell on the techniques of running but there are a number of basic points to bear in mind. First remember you're not running so as to be a good runner. What I mean is that technique is important, but not critical. If bad technique means you work harder that's no loss, particularly in relation to what we're looking for. Learn to relax, especially in your distance work, as any tension will be magnified after a few miles.

Try and achieve a good stride length, so that you have to use your muscles in pulling back as you stride through, but, bear in mind, that if you over-reach you get 'retardation'. This means that when your feet hit the floor, you're basically stopping yourself, because your bodyweight is back too far. Try and put some spring into your stride so that your natural momentum puts your weight over your leg by the time it touches the floor and you're then ready to 'pull through' your stride. If you do this, your bodyweight, particularly if you are heavy, should not be a problem.

As I've said previously, I run on the balls of my feet. I avoid running flat-footed unless going downhill. I run on the balls of my feet for two reasons. Firstly, I build up my calves - particularly when hill-sprinting and secondly, by being on my toes or ball of the foot, I can get a more natural spring into my stride. Also I find I can change pace quickly if I'm changing from a jog to a sprint - say between lamp-posts if I'm running a 'Fartlek' programme. I build my calves up so that I have better stability and mobility for other work, as I have stronger lower legs and ankles.

I also always endeavour to make the best use of my arms. Keep your shoulders loose and get a reasonable swing in front. When you're sprinting your arms do as much work as your legs. Your arms, when you sprint, set the pace for your legs and particularly when you hill-sprint, your arms become central, because you throw your arms up high which lifts your whole body and allows your knee to come up high on the hill. It is quite possible to hill-sprint with no knee-lift, but for me you're defeating the object of the exercise. By lifting the knee, you increase the workout, so making the exercise more difficult and you also strengthen the muscles responsible for lifting your legs, which greatly enhances your kicking ability.

High Knee Lifts
This reaches it's ultimate in the 'high knee lift' training exercises, where your arms are thrown skyward and your knees propelled high into the chest. When practising High Knees, you 'stab' your feet into the ground and advance only a few inches with each stride - so much so, that a sprint which would normally be covered in 15 strides, should take 50/60 strides of High Knee lifts - a real cracker!

When hill-sprinting on my own, I start with a few short-step high knee lifts before I get into the stride. This gives me some initial momentum, gets me into the leg and arm action and achieves movement without exerting the huge strain that can be applied if you simply explode into a long stride on the hill. Unfortunately, when sprinting competitively against someone, the luxury of this easy start is impossible.

When I'm hill sprinting, I'll alter the stride length - sometimes I'll do short, fast, stabbing steps to work leg speed and other times I'll lengthen the stride to the maximum possible, given the angle of the hill, to get more of a pulling effort which strengthens the upper hamstrings and glutes.

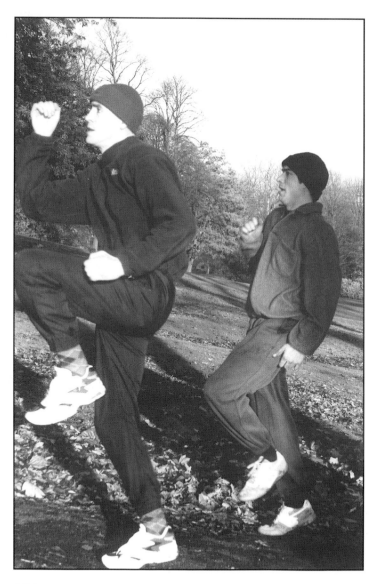

High Knee Lifts - made even harder here, by doing them on an incline. Never make this exercise competitive, as there should be no race.

Technical Tip.

If you're having to sprint against your training partners, then some technique improvement is advisable. The best sprinters are those who make it look easy and herein lies the key. Even the most powerful of sprinters seemingly control the input of power by keeping relaxed and appearing to glide and Michael Johnson must be the ultimate example of that. What kills smoothness is 'tightening up' - keep your form and mental focus within your own self, even when someone's coming up behind to overtake you. Don't get mentally side-tracked by concentrating on them and don't force your efforts - just keep a good leg and arm cadence and try to maintain your leg and arm pace and never force a hard increase of effort.

I remember reading a book by Herschel Walker, a very successful American pro-footballer, who said try sprinting with a handful of tacks - if you tense up, you'll know about it! Your speed is essentially dependent upon two factors, stride length and stride speed or frequency. That having been said, if the end result was simply a product of just these two factors, the fastest and strongest should win every time and we know that just isn't the case. The biomechanical factors often take a back seat to many of the psychological and motivational factors. Remember the sprint work I'm advocating is not an end in itself and perfect technique is not a pre-requisite for achieving good results from the effort. I'm not out to win races, rather from sprinting I want to develop explosive power, leg strength and ability to achieve hard set goals based on time or distance.

Finally on technique, try to keep your legs ie. toes and knees pointing straight forward, not letting your feet fall too wide of an imaginary line, otherwise your motion forward will be crab-like. You hands should piston vertically up and down and not cross your body, which will throw you off balance. Unless you are practising exaggerated 'high knee lifts', do not let your hands so much higher than your head.

Adding Weight

Tremendous gains can be made by the addition of weights to your sprint training. Many years ago I acquired wrist/ankle weights with velcro fastenings that I've used for punching and leg exercises and also for running. They only weigh a couple of pounds each, but when you're having to move them at speed, the extra weight soon makes a telling difference. I used to wear them as ankle weights, but the additional impact and knee strain was counter-productive. Since then I restricted them to the wrists and the effect on both performance and the arms is marked.

A small 20 litre day sac, the sort used for the long fell events is ideal to run with. Over long distances the pack is comfortable and you can get into a good stride pattern, although it doesn't work as well for sprinting. What you can acquire from an ex-army surplus shop is the older and heavy American flak jacket. It's a sleeveless waistcoat and weighs in the region of 20lbs. It fits well and you can sprint effectively in one.

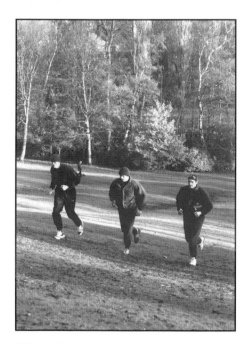

Hill work - the first easy sprint to stretch the legs, muscles and tendons.

Hill Work

With hill work scenery is unimportant - whether you're on a grass slope or tarmac you are going to feel too distressed to bother about the scenery or your boredom threshold. If you are on the road doing it, pick somewhere where you're not waiting for people to get out of the way. If it's a steep hill and they're old and going up, it could take forever. Decide what you are going to do before you get there and vary the routine. You will never feel consistently the same and setting too high goals on every occasion is wrong - **'know your body, but ignore you're mind'**. My specific hill programme is described in the chapter on single person drills and whether you are on your own or with others, hills must be included.

Once you start to work your hill sprints, you'll find that speed is no longer a factor and your technique will change accordingly. The hill is the weight handicap. I've no way of equating inclines to resultant degrees of physical output, but only a few degrees of hill must equate to sprinting on the flat with 10/20lbs extra. It probably gives the greatest degree of satisfaction in achieving a hill sprint session properly, than any other running exercise. You can incorporate variations such as 'high knee lifts' in hill work.

Step or Stair Work
The last area of sprint work I want to cover is 'step work'. Over the years of training I've been reasonably lucky at being able to find areas near where I've lived that have had suitable steps aeither in public parks or in hilly residential areas. On the video 'Fit To Fight' in the Pavement Arena series we shot part of the video at one of my old, favourite locations. This was in Manchester and was one of the most ideal locations for hill and step work.

I probably dislike running as much today as I have for the past couple of decades and more. It's the boredom. Running brings home to me the very clear fact that I have a short attention span. Often on a longish run I stop - not because of stress or fatigue, but simply boredom. There have been times, however, when I've set out on a run and my spirits have soared and I know then, quite dramatically, that training equates to freedom. During a two year sojourn high up on the North West coast of Scotland some years back, one of my training runs took me along a coast road. As it happened I lived on the coast road so either direction took me by the sea and running there wasn't hard. At times, however, a 40mph wind in the face made you feel as if you were running against a Sumo wrestler, but bored I wasn't.

I now live again in a city conurbation and running in the streets is hard. If I add up my mileage, currently I put in twice the distance on the treadmill as I do on the road.

Some people are mentally cut out for distance work and that's good, but as you have probably gathered by now it's not distance work that will contribute to our success in a combat or conflict situation.

Machine Running

First, find a gym that is equipped with running treadmills that will incline under power, so you can vary all three factors just as you would in the street ie **Time, Distance, Incline.** Ignore the machines time to distance ratio as I find these woefully inaccurate, but it doesn't matter as you are after effect not completion of a distance. The target should be a time one, balanced against output of effort. Whether it accurately measures that you are doing 6 miles per hour is irrelevant just so long as you're stretched.

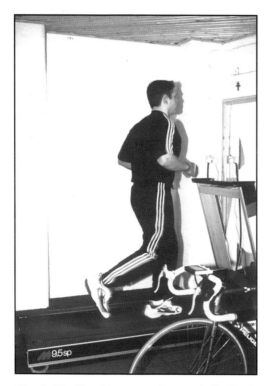

Treadmill - like this one, make sure it 'inclines' under power, so you can always use it to run uphill. They are usually fast enough to sustain a sprint to exhaustion or a long push.

My sessions in the 'aerobic' room in the gym are often not!. By that I mean that my sessions often become very anaerobic in nature. This could be on the treadmill, bike, rower, or any other piece of equipment, but sometimes I'll use them for 'long-slow-distance work when necessary.

Other times I'll duplicate the outdoors hill work by putting in heavy, steep angle sprints to failure. Mainly, however, I'll try to sustain a 'heavy push', at a good pace, on a taxing incline for as long as possible. Often I'll use a Walkman and try to keep my concentration focussed on the effort and not let it drift. You can mix, say, 2 pieces of equipment on a 15/20 minute rotation on each, or a 20 minute machine session and a 20 minute bagwork/skipping session. Over a 20 minute period, on an inclined treadmill you can come off it exhausted. For me, they are one of the best 'standby' pieces of equipment there is. That's not to decry any other CV kit, because I use them all, but I'll always gravitate first to a treadmill.

Where To Run

Depending on your domestic location, this may not be that flexible. For me, it's easier to say where not to run and that's on the roads. The reason is not because of the hard surfaces, as they can mitigated by good footwear, predominantly it's the poor air quality we face. Sulphur dioxide, ozone, carbon monoxide and other pollutants, all have a detrimental effect on our health and wellbeing. Increases in child and adult asthma are all being attributed to increases in pollution. Particulates in the air can clog up lungs from such sources as pollen, dust, smoke and even rubber from car tyres.

Probably the biggest single problem is carbon monoxide. It can, at its worst, asphyxiate, but in moderate amounts, which we will inhale whilst running in heavy or moderate traffic, it is still dangerous. Carbon monoxide inhibits oxygen delivery to the cells and can cause weakness, dizziness and nausea. It's effects are increased with particular weather conditions, particularly if foggy or in still, hot environments. Hot summer days, in a built-up and traffic-heavy industrial area, can be a bad combination for anyone, but particularly for those people who have any pre-disposition to chest problems or allergies such as hayfever. If you do, switch to machine work indoors or switch to a park or rural environment, even if it means a drive to get there.

I know from bitter personal experience, how demoralising and debilitating hayfever can be, particularly in a city environment. In some extremely bad conditions, running less than a mile will be all I can manage. At times like these, you must accept the inevitable and not push it, which will cause stress and strains to your heart. Make changes to your programme, move indoors to CV equipment and improvise.

CHAPTER 6

WEIGHTS

Like running, I started using weights in my youth and equally like running, weights for me, are not an end in themselves. Like all my 'support training' I am not driven to achieve great results and I have limited aims which relate to my overall goal which is physical maintenance to practise martial arts and constant readiness for combat.

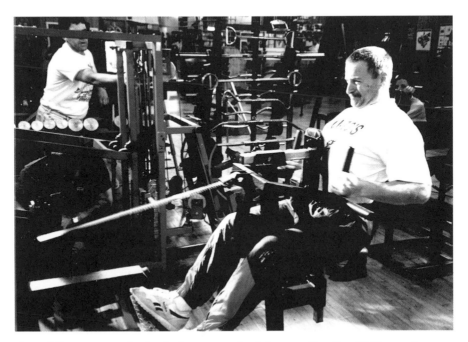

Seated Row - a must for developing a strong back for grappling. Ian McCranor, former England Karate International and doorman, knows the necessity of working with weights.

Weight training is invaluable for over 50% of that readiness. In a fight, size and strength will count. Muscle is armour plate and helps resist blows and is the basis of power. Having said that, maybe only some 20%, as I believe strength and power are two separate things. Power for me means impact and I've seen 18 stone bodybuilders who can't impact when put on pads or a bag and they may even be working the doors!. POWER IS STRENGTH ON THE MOVE. It demands technique, explosiveness, relaxation and the application of body dynamics to gain a ballistic effect (see 'Powerstrike').

As the years go by, weights, to me, become increasingly important and takes up more training time in percentage terms than ever before. As bone density and muscle strength lessen with age, training with weights provides the compensatory effect. It strengthens joints and tendons, in my case, stressed and worn by 32 years of martial arts. The fact I'm fit, flexible and powerful is due in no small part to years of weights. Note that I omitted 'strong' from the above list of my gains from weights as this is even more subjective and less of benefit to me. The beneficial effect on joints, tendons, muscles and connective tissue cannot be underestimated and anyone who has an interest in their ability to survive combat or conflict, must have a weights programme.

In nearly every chapter, I apologise for what this book is not about and I'll do it again - this book is not about weight training and the technique of specific exercises. Any of the bodybuilding - weights magazines all have excellent articles, which over a period give you all the possible variations on a theme of training routines you could want. You will have to decide on a programme which satisfies your personal requirements, accepting that over a period, these will change.

Many of the factors which affect the decision on a particular weights programme are to do with physical stature. Again, I don't want to go into an exposition of the 3, broad physical types we are told the human race divides into, that is Endomorph, Ectomorph and Mesomorph, but how we are naturally built will determine our approach to a weights programme.

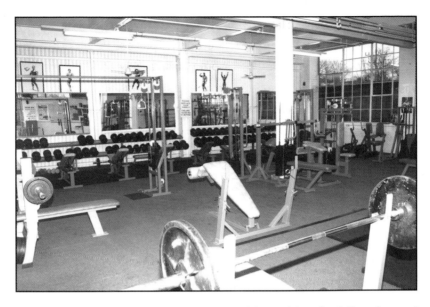

A well-equipped weights gym. A wide range of free weights, dumbells and a good variety of machines (Sporting Bodies - Wakefield).

In the '70's when I was 'working the doors' in Manchester and at which time I won the 'British Middleweight' Full Contact title, I weighed marginally over 11.5 stones. Now I have an additional 3 stones on top of that and over the years, my approach to how I train with weights has varied. If you want to put weight on, then like all training - 'less is more'. You need to keep the reps down and the weight up. Keep the exercises basic and forget putting a great number of variations into the routine, which only work the finer points of muscle development.

It might be, that as you get into weights, your attitude changes and it becomes an all-consuming passion and takes on more of an end in itself. Whatever the motivation or end goal, it should be approached properly. Know what you are doing, get advice, try and train with someone who knows what they're doing and don't deceive yourself about what you think you can lift. I'll keep saying it 'til I'm blue in the face - Power is not solely a function of strength. Don't think because you can heave heavy weights in all directions, that you'll be able to kick and punch hard - you won't!, but 'base strength' is the basis for the overall framework of what you are going to do with combative technique.

Don't believe the bollocks about heavy muscles slowing you down. Tell martial artists like Terry O'Neill, or a sprinter like Linford Christie that weight training and good musculature will slow you down. As always it's the people who HAVEN'T and CAN'T that tell you, you SHOULDN'T. Let me tell you, if I had the choice to fight one of two people, both with equal technique, bottle, aggression and ability, I'll pick the 10 stone one to go at, not the one weighing in at 20 stones - size, strength and weight count - anyone tells you different, it's bollocks.

One good way that I saw the various factors of weight training represented was as follows:-

1. Training session length

2. Training session frequency.

3. Body part training frequency.

4. Exercise selection and performance.

5. Repetition speed.

6. Training session volume and intensity.

7. Weight and reps.

8. Rest intervals between sets.

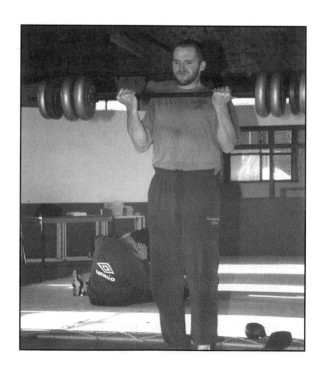

Curls, in the dojo, after a hard Karate session with reps to failure over 4 sets and a medium weight.

High Volume? - Low Volume 'Heavy? The argument rages on and isn't a suitable topic for this book. What I would say, however, is that for a combative approach to training, we need as much as anything, a programme which satisfies our subjective mental demands. Many of these are dictated by our current, motivational factors. If such issues as 'confidence' is, we believe, built by simply being 'big', our training will incline towards that. Doormen, as a breed, very often train for size and consequent strength, particularly when other combative skills are absent. They seldom train for muscular endurance.

Over an 8-year period, when I worked the doors in Manchester, size alone could never be a sole factor, given the range and intensity of cardio-vascular training and martial arts, particularly inclined towards competition. The weight training at that time was slanted towards a muscle stamina and the intensity was through volume, not of weight, but of repetitions of weight. Now, I'm less overly concerned with muscle stamina and probably strike a somewhat better balance.

If you have a good CV regime, then you can afford to cut back on the reps and increase the weight. Lean muscle growth is always difficult, particularly with a high aerobic output, as a loss of muscle mass can often occur. Before we leave the foggy arena of low or high volume weight training, it would seem that our **Growth Hormone (GH)** is, in fact, most effectively stimulated by high volume training - strange eh! High volume is broadly described as lifting loads of 50-60% of maximum, with high sets and reps.

GH is a major feature in the effective protein 'take-up', body fat breakdown and general regulator of body metabolism. Also GH would seem to have an ability to enhance the liver's output of glucose (blood sugar), whilst, at the same time, reducing glycogen uptake by the cells, for energy. The result is that glycogen is stored for longer and the body will have to utilise fat for energy. More reps - higher volume would appear to set GH off.

CV Endurance
Don't ignore using a weights programme for cardiovascular endurance. It is possible to put aerobics and weights together to build endurance, but what has to be recognised, is that simply extending the traditional way of working with weights won't work, ie simply doing 40 reps of bench press instead of the usual 8 - 10.

The emphasis has to change in that the target base has to be a time one eg. 30 - 45 seconds of an exercise, with a weight of approx. 40 - 60% of your 1 rep max. Time then also comes into the rest period, which should be within the 15 - 20 sec arena, ie. enough time to get to the next exercise or piece of equipment.

The 'circuit' which is what is built up, may have 10 - 12 stations or less and ideally, the variety of exercises will alternately hit upper and lower body. Completion of one circuit is basically one set, which could be repeated 3 - 4 times. To obtain some variety, you could alter the circuit on each set or keep it the same. Alternatively, circuits could be changed on different days of the week.

The weights circuit, has developed to a very sophisticated degree, particularly in the United States. After a heavy exercise on the weights, the next 'stance' would be an aerobic exercise eg. stationary bike, skipping, jogging on the spot, star jumps etc, but anything to keep you moving. A variation on this type of training was that which developed in Scandinavia called PHA (Peripheral Heart Action). This gave no rest between say 4 weight routines, with 20 reps plus in each set. At the end of the 4, a rest could be taken only briefly and not so the heart rate ever fell below 120bpm.

You can construct your own PACE GYM, although the proper PACE equipment is specifically designed for weights-based CV circuits.

So what exercises do we need for what we want to achieve? Are there any muscle groups we should emphasise and are there any muscle groups we don't need to work? Unfortunately, for those looking for an easy option, the answer to the latter is no. We need every muscle group to give an all-round combative ability and we therefore can't omit anything from our programme, ranging from a strong grip, to a strong back for pulling, chest and shoulders for pushing and legs for stability and strength to resist when pushing and pulling. And, certainly not to be forgotten, to run with.

You can't escape any muscle group however hard and however difficult it might be to see gains. Broadly, you can break your body into workable parts, chest, back, shoulders, arms, legs and abs. Seems simple so far, but now we enter the world of complexity of combining muscle groups into workouts and then further sub-dividing the work for these muscle groups into various exercises and then how many times an exercise is repeated ie set and then how many repetitions of that particular movement we will do in each set and the percentage of our maximum that we will lift. It is down to purely personal choice and preference as to

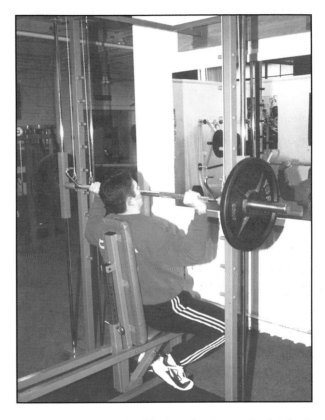

Seated Press on the 'Smith'. A good strict exercise for shoulders and upper pecs. Sometimes pressing behind the neck can cause shoulder problems.

how long it takes us to complete a cycle. Over the years I've tried everything, particularly as I'm as susceptible to a well-reasoned argument about the benefits of one programme over another as the next man. In reality, it probably doesn't matter. If after a weights session you've pushed, pulled and lifted 20,000 pounds approx. of weight, you're achieving results, whatever programme you've followed. The one that works for me, probably more in terms of comfort, is to keep major body parts away from each other. What I mean by this is that I won't work chest with back or back with shoulders or chest with a full leg workout.

I'm going to get under weights some four and possibly five times a week if I'm in the U.K. and maybe only 3 if I'm abroad or away and I can find a gym. As a working

Bodyguard, I don't always maintain the consistency I want, but wherever I am I'll compensate with increasing the other work eg. running or working against my own bodyweight. A weights cycle for me would be, say, to start with chest, during which session I'd put in biceps and possibly calves. Sit-ups and other abdominal work happens on every session irrespective of what I'm doing.

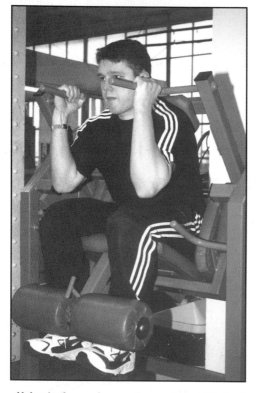

Abdominal crunches on the machine - it's hard to cheat on this, but I've seen it done.

The next visit would be to work back, another 'major muscle' group with triceps, hamstrings and abs and the third part of the cycle would be shoulders with front thighs and probably calves again. Every session would finish with abs and most sessions would start with 20 or more minutes in the aerobics room on equipment or in the bag room. If my main session on the weights is going to be legs and a hard session, it will only be twenty minutes and I won't allow this aerobics part to turn into a heavy anaerobic session on the bike or treadmill. It is probably not advisable to mix 'major' muscle groups in one session. Keep chest, legs and back separate. You may want to include a partial leg workout with any muscle group, but limit your time in the gym and see how it all works out for you personally.

You can put traps into either the shoulder or back routine and forearms into one of the others. On a personal front, I don't use wrist straps as I don't want to be training with weights my wrists can't handle. I don't want to reduce the degree of difficulty in being able to push up and control the weight with my grip, particularly on exercises like chins. Anyone whose tried to scale a climbing wall or rockface knows the advantage of a strong grip and strong fingers. If I can't support my own body weight for 10 chins with my own grip, I'm either overweight or my grip is too weak.

Many times when working the doors, my grip saved me and helped me control a situation, particularly when I had those rare opportunities to get someone by the throat. Judo men know the value of forearm strength and if you look at a Judoka's forearms you'll know what I mean.

Broadly, and this is purely a personal preference, I work to a measured combination of 3 sets per exercise, per muscle group, where the first set is the lightest and acts as a warm-up set of maybe 12 reps and with the second being as heavy as I can go without any 'cheating'. The third set may be somewhat lighter with an extra two reps over the second set or I may keep the weight the same and try for the same reps.

I've no argument with 'cheating' as a technique, as advocated by some of the most experienced and biggest bodybuilders and I know it is effective, however, it simply doesn't suit me mentally. I want to stay as strict as possible and get my eventual power from else-where. Also, unfortunately, many people simply copy a 'cheat' technique for every-thing they do in the gym and wonder why they make no gains.

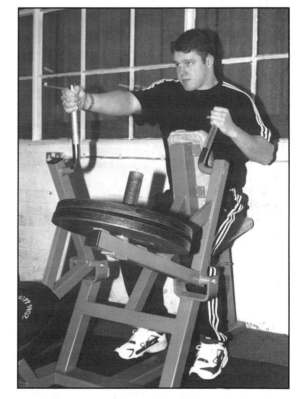

As with many weight training exercises, such as Hammer Rows, you can see the combative benefit.

Some people train with weights which are probably double the amount they should work with if they were strict.

How many exercises you want to do for each broad muscle group is one of personal preference. Suffice it to say that there are more than enough variations to keep anyone from being bored. Vary your routines in respect of the exercises you do. Your muscles need to be shocked into growth from the complacency of an unaltered, over-regular routine. It might work for you to go 'heavy' on chest say and the next lighten the load a bit and increase the effort by increasing the reps. More reps increase 'muscle stamina' as well as strength, but may not help in putting on size or muscle density. There are opposing schools of thought on this and I don't want to fall down, on either side of the argument, as both approaches have merit from a 'combative' requirement.

Remember though, that it in a conflict situation, where, as everyone says *"my muscles turned to water"*, strength may not be enough - the effects of mild psychological shock which has the over-compensation of drawing blood to the core and away from the body's periphery - deprives the muscles of their working energy source. Explosive power now takes over for fight or flight and this is a consequence of technique, training, mental aggression and a correct approach to being first in the fight ie. pre-emptive.

Choose a gym which seems to have a good balance between free weights and machines. Choose a gym which maintains its equipment and is prepared to re-invest in new kit which it feels appropriate. An up-market, machine-only, cv inclined operation is okay, but the emphasis is wrong for what we want to achieve. Don't get me wrong, when I'm working away either in the U.K. or abroad, I'm grateful for any gym in the hotel and, for example, the Radisson in Moscow has one of the best gyms I've found in all of the former Soviet Union. An experienced trainer can make do with very little, but don't set out looking for very little.

Legs

Its appropriate to stress the importance of leg work. Legs - I've heard it said that "legs are the second heart". Unfortunately, legs are the first things which go under stress. We've all been in situations where we've said afterwards that our legs went, be it fear, shock, surprise, sudden activity, stress. This always seems strange, given that our legs contain some of the most powerful muscles in the body.

Muscles such as the quadriceps, which are responsible for straightening the legs and which can support a tonnage of several times the weight of the person. Their antagonists are the bicep femoris, or as we more commonly know them - the hamstrings. They are activated whenever you raise your heel ie. walking, running etc. Finally, the calves or gastrocnemius, engaged whenever you extend your toe to the floor and underneath lies the soleus, which extends the foot, primarily, when the knee is flexed to a position of 90 degrees or more.

The legs are activated repeatedly and place huge demands on the body's cardiovascular system and the whole of the CNS - not equalled by the upper body. As is the case with all muscles, if the demand is adequately intense, the CNS will supply the answer in the form of muscular overcompensation - in other words, bigger muscles.

What we should know, however, is also the fact that CNS induced growth is not exclusively muscle specific. What this means is that the

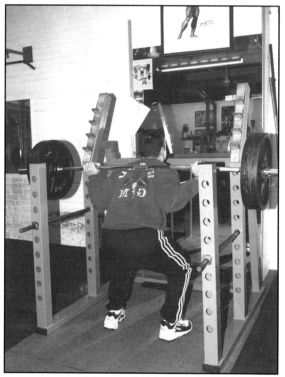

The Squat - basic, strict and heavy. It is acknowledged that this exercise has a 'whole body' effect in growth terms.

adaptive response will not just take place in the leg area, but will happen in lesser, but involved body parts. This is known as the 'indirect adaptive effect'. The bigger the muscle groups activated, the bigger the adaptive response. This is why so many schools of thought recommend squats as one of the finest bodybuilding exercises in its own right. It would seem that during squats, some 14 muscle groups are involved.

It is now a commonly held view that a 'heavy' squat routine will have a total body effect. I suffer, marginally, from knee problems, particularly with free squats and have to make do with either a 'Smith' machine or a leg press. Whilst some people swear by the effects of a leg press machine, it does not quite match the results you'll get from a free squat. There is also a tendency by people to overload the leg press and 'squat' for three-four inches, if that. The movement still needs to be full.

I've always found it difficult to build leg size due to the other CV work and also kicking, but so long as you know your legs won't ever let you down, then the size is of lesser importance.

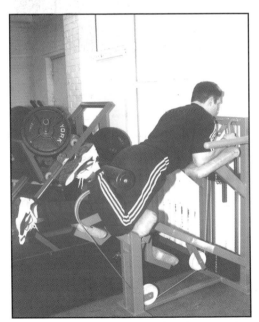

Single leg hamstring curl - designed so as to isolate the leg and prevent cheating.

Look at the legs of tennis players. Most look like they've been on a heavy weights programme. Whilst many do, these days, train with weights, the size is mainly a product of the explosive 'shuttle work' they do across the court. Tennis players have a good VO_2max and in the shuttle 'beep' tests, score one of the highest levels before they go 'anaerobic'. If you get the opportunity, try and do a 25 metre 'beep' test and see how you fair. As the pace picks up, you are sprinting from one side of the hall to another, but remember, what becomes an anaerobic sprint to you, is still, as with the tennis players, probably a comfortable jog.

This is what we want to achieve with our legs - the ability to carry on. As a consequence, it may be that our weights programme for legs should be geared to 'high output' ie. more reps in the 20+ region for each set. I read an article which was an interview with **Steve Reeves**, who at the time was in his '60s and trained regularly. His leg workout was 1,000 continuous reps on the leg press machine (with a weight that would have stumped me after 25 reps!). He'd take years to build up to that level - the interviewer watched him do it by the way!

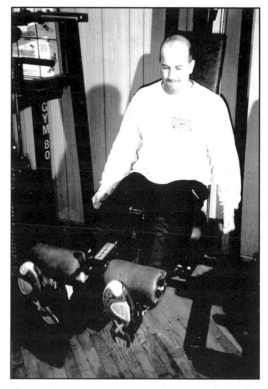

Certainly not your archetypal tennis player, but Geoff, after years of Coventry door work, knows the important of building muscle endurance in the legs - not just stamina.

He also cycled up an 11-mile hill, almost flat out and used to describe passing people half his age who couldn't keep up. His mental strength and focus was awesome, but over the years he had moved the emphasis from pure strength and bodybuilding to muscle endurance. He was still big, even with that level of output, but more importantly, he could carry on with a high level of intense effort, without reaching an anaerobic intolerance. Be quite clear though, about what you want to achieve.

My objectives are:- **Muscle Endurance , Muscle Strength, Cardio-Vascular Capacity, Anaerobic/Lactic Fuel Tolerance** and lastly, **Maintenance of Skill and Combative Willpower.**

If you combine weights and aerobic training, then do the weights first if you want to lose fat. The reasoning behind this is that the weights being anaerobic will cause your muscles to 'burn up' local glycogen stores by as much as 50%. This means that when you get to the anaerobic training, you will much sooner be utilising stored fat for fuel.

Combining training routines or 'cross training' as we have come to know it, is a skill in itself, even before we begin to train in our combative skills. A high level of fitness is the essential ingredient of any combat environment. When the action starts, you will go from anaerobic to lactic in a matter of seconds. If you have not prepared for this, you will fail at your task, particularly if the fear, shock of the event and psychological stress is high. Under these conditions, skills and techniques which are not ingrained and supported by fitness will fail.

Fat Loss Through Muscle Gain

Don't just think that you will only lose weight (fat) through aerobic exercise - muscles burn fat! Being in possession of lean muscle mass will in itself burn calories - in fact, one pound of muscle will burn between 50 - 100 calories at rest per day. If you could put on 5lbs of additional muscle, you would burn anywhere from 250 - 500 calories extra each day.

CHAPTER 7

SINGLE DRILLS

Often we are unable to train with the benefit of others and also, particularly in my case, when abroad or away, unable to find a gym. There are a number of standby exercises which we can resort to, not least of these being to run.

Recently working in the Algerian desert, I was up at 0545 and out running around the mixed dust and tarmac of the compound we were in. It was approx 650 meters in a rectangular shape and my routine was 4/5 laps, building up the pace for a last lap blast and then onto a concrete basketball pitch for sets of skipping, shuttle sprints, shadow boxing and kicking and then back to my room for sets of press-ups and sit-ups. I was back in my room by 0630 with 10 mins for the strength work. By that time it was starting to get hot, but a cool breeze, the sun coming up and the ubiquitous Walkman kept me going through the boredom of running in circles. Daytime temperatures reached in excess of 100 degrees and made it impossible to train any other time.

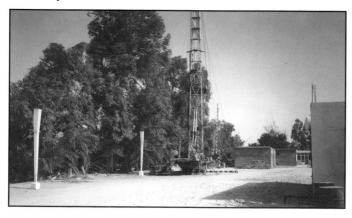

The compound in Algeria - not an inviting place to train - but it still has to be done.

In the absence of a punch bag this was a balanced 'circuit'. Time was not on my side. I couldn't get up any earlier as it was dark and the Algerian army guards, who were on patrol during the night, were not a body of men in whom I ever had confidence in their ability to distinguish friend from foe. First light seemed the safest time. I was constrained at the other end by the requirement to get ready, breakfast and start work, but if more time had been available I would have increased both the run, by the addition of one more circuit and then added some squat thrusts and the like whilst on the basketball court. A Gatorade mix was essential, both pre, during and after this workout.

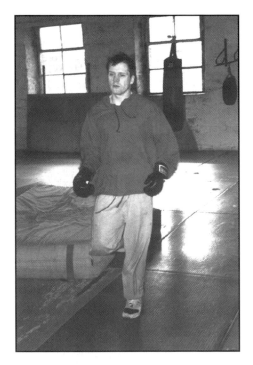

*Solo **wind sprints** across the dojo, during a martial arts session.*

Running

In the Chapter on running I've more than adequately expressed my somewhat 'love/hate' relationship that I've had with running, but it is still one of the best ways, in the absence of a well equipped CV gym to keep fit. I've also described the variations of running and in this book we can find enough to keep us occupied either when with partners or on our own.

Hill Work

The photographs on these pages show my current hill. I use both the grass and two paths that flank it. I start with a half mile warm-up - stretch out at the bottom of the hill and then set off on the first sprint at an average pace. It should be taxing but not overly fast.

Stage 1
Stretch Out

The object of the first one should be to acquaint the knees, tendons and muscles to the incline, the arms pumping and to break past that first breathing or more correctly, breathless, barrier. My time on that first sprint is approx. 1.25 minutes. I walk back down because I want to get the most out of each one and in this exercise, recovery is important.

Long Stride

At the bottom I turn straight back and set off again, noting the time. On this repetition, I am after as long a stride pattern as possible and try to pull myself up the hill with long pulls reaching far forward with each step. This should also be faster than the first sprint, but will not be the fastest as, on a hill, a long stride actually retards forward momentum, but the object in getting the stride length is for power building. We are less concerned with adhering to perfect technique.

Fastest time! - all out on the last sprint on the grass - it's a total burn at the end.

Fastest Time

Back down again and then the third and maybe last one on the grass is the fastest all out. This asks for as fast a leg frequency as possible, shorter strides and a higher knee action, with the stride simply being sufficient to meet the angle of hill that's coming towards you. The arm action is higher than you

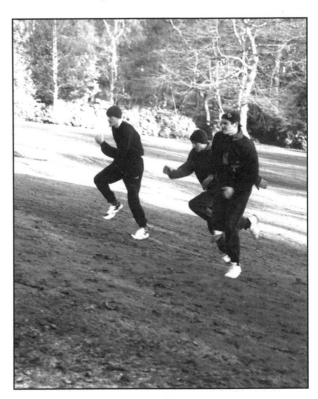

would use on the flat as you are attempting to 'throw' yourself up the hill. This should be the most demanding of the three reps but it is over the quickest. Recovery after this one will need to be longer.

Stage 2

From here I move onto the path where the pace will be faster as there is more spring from the tarmac and often a wet and soggy grass slope can make obtaining a grip hard and spring difficult, but this all goes towards the effort. Now, different from the long grass slope, I vary both the technique and now the distance! I don't keep to the long distance on each sprint as the lactic acid build up is now too debilitating for the longer effort.

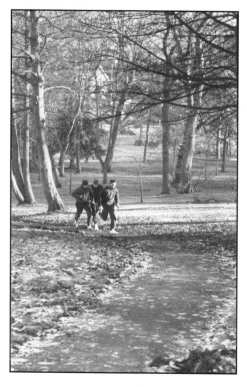

Stage 2 - now onto the 'tarmac' path at the side of the grass slope. This is for shorter, faster sprints, with more spring off the harder sur-

Long Push

My first rep is from the very bottom and go for a long pull at a medium pace. The build up of lactic acid makes it now impossible to go for total speed at this distance - it's a 'push', but not all out.

Short Sprints

After this I then move the starting point up the path and vary the speed and stride length as I did before, finishing with a blast over 40 or so metres. By this time you shouldn't be able to stand without wobbling. Usually, there are just 3 sprints in total on this tarmac path.

Stage 3

After this I traverse warily and wobbly across the grass slope to a shallower angled roadway and work another 3/4 reps, of which 2 will be backwards sprints.

These are excellent for building the front thighs and are, to say the least, extremely taxing. Always pick a quiet, even, straight path for these, because you don't want to be looking backwards as you sprint. You use no knee lift, simply reach well behind with each stride and use your arms in a cross-body action so as to allow your hips to roll from side to side, which brings your legs in a somewhat long circular action. It has a devastating effect on your quads.

As we were not designed to run or walk backwards, it takes a higher degree of effort to go in reverse. Tests have shown that a 4 mile per hour walk forward on a treadmill, which raises the heart to 106 bpm, will be boosted to in excess of 150 bpm when done backwards.

Running is similarly affected - VO_2 max is up from 60% to 84% when running and the heart rate up from 151 to over 170 bpm. Its excellent for the quads.

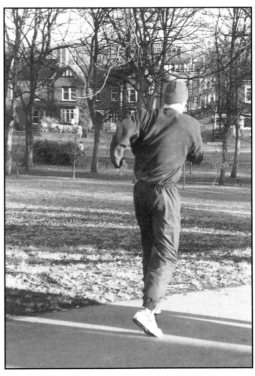

Stage 4

Finally, it's 2 reps of high knee lifts. At the end of a hard session, these will finish you lungs and

Stage 3 - backward hill sprints. One of the best quad builders, but always use a hill. Any steepness of hill will do, but vary the distance - always go for your fastest pace. With a partner, you can race.

legs off. The technique takes some getting used to and will only work if you lean back. By doing this, you allow the maximum potential for leg lift. Your knees are pumped vertically very high with each stroke, probably only covering some 12 inches over the ground with each stride. If you actually feel you are going nowhere, then you're doing it right. This is all enabled by an exaggerated arm action, which you pump high in the air to raise your body off the ground. Never use too steep a

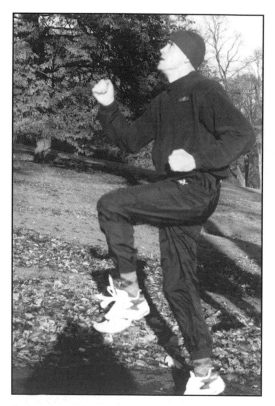

Stage 4 - high knee lifts on the hill. If you had anything left, these should finish you off. After these, it's a wobble back to the car, which, if you've any sense, should be waiting for you at the bottom of the hill.

hill and if you're really tired by this stage, then work on the flat, 15 - 20 metres is sufficient and you'll probably take 60 steps to cover this distance. This exercise as with all the hill work can be incorporated in 'Partner Drills'

I'll have a mix of fluid replacement drink such as 'Power Blast' with me, which I will have spread over the whole session, having had some prior and enough left for after the workout. I'll have paced it's intake over the session. It's over, as a session, depending on the length of rest periods in about 25 minutes, but it feels like you've been at it for 2 hours.

Skipping

I persevered with skipping for a long time, before I was halfway competent enough to get any beneficial effect from it. Having got to that point, it's one of the mainstays in my gym work when I'm on my own. As with all exercises, you dictate the pace and intensity of what you do, and skipping is no exception. We're told that skipping can equal running in its effective calorific burn, but to me that's meaningless. A 'hard' skipping routine for 2-3 minutes can leave you anaerobic and gasping for breath. Mix high knee lifts into it and very soon you're feeling the lactic acid build-up in your quads.

Also, apart from walking up a steep mountain with a 60lb pack on your back, skipping has to be one of the best calf exercises there is. It's plyometric benefits are obvious, but less obvious is the fact it builds, not only agility but good lower leg muscle control. I've watched people in competition who obviously lack calf and ankle strength and who seem 'flat footed'. It's hard to describe but it's one of those things, as they say - 'you'll know it when you see it'.

Good calves mean good balance, sound footing and explosiveness. They provide that initial spring and explosion linked with a driving power in the quads. Whenever I get the rare opportunity to be in the hills these days, I realise how weak my ankles are as I negotiate rough ground, but 'muscle memory' eventually comes to my aid and I get into the groove again and feel a degree of agility and balance come back into the lower legs.

I've used skipping as one of my main methods of warming up before stretching. I keep the intensity low for this and make it last for at least 3-5 minutes, then stretch - in particular the shoulder joints if you're going onto the bag. Below in the specific section on Bag Work, I've described how I increase the intensity by combining skipping with both the bag and punching.

You can make skipping as hard or as easy as you want. It can be long and slow, to stay aerobic or, you can increase the pace and the degree of difficulty to stretch your aerobic threshold to the point of being anaerobic.

Skipping is also safe, because the impact is 'low', as defined by today's somewhat arbitrary 'fitness professional' definition. An extra-heavy rope or added weights has been proved to develop muscle mass and compliments a strength development programme. That having been said, it's primary benefit is aerobic and with a skipping rope, you can develop 2 of the key components to physical fitness - development of the cardio-vascular and respiratory systems.

Technical Tip

Start skipping by simply doing alternate steps over the rope ie. one circuit of the rope with one step over it with one foot, then the other. Don't start by jumping both feet over at the same time. It's actually a lot harder and more tiring and also makes it more difficult to expand into more difficult steps.

Keep the arms bent sufficient to allow the rope to just skim the floor. Eventually, you can skip with the rope just missing the floor, but this is pushing things a bit too much, too soon. Try and use your wrists to do the work - skipping has a great effect on the forearms by the way.

As the rope completes its circle, make sure it touches the floor underneath you. This may sound obvious but it's not. Many people who start skipping hold their hands too far in front of their body and the circle of the rope is completed at the bottom of the cycle, too far in front of the feet. This causes the rope to 'bounce' off the floor and into the front of the feet. Keep your shoulders and elbows back.

When you feel comfortable and can go for longer than a minute without getting tied up, it's up to you to experiment. Try and watch experts skip, even an 18 stone super-heavyweight boxer seems as light as a 7 stone girl gymnast when it comes to skipping. Stay 'light on the feet' and try out some patterns for yourself.

One-Leg Hops (Skipping)

Try one-legged hops for a count of 20-25 - this is a real calf-building exercise. You may have to work up to this number but whatever target you set yourself, when you've finished the single leg skips, change to the other leg and repeat. You won't do many, as the muscle effort to give that 'plyometric' spring required in the calf is substantial. Also, try 'tracking' forward and backward, not just on the spot.

High Knee Lift (Skipping)

Again, if you're looking for intensity out of a skipping routine, high knee lifts are one of the best. Hopefully, the following description as to how to do this won't confuse you beyond all reason. The technique is not to do a high lift on each step. Rather it involves a double hop on each leg.

A single hop does not buy sufficient time for the other leg to reach any height in the knee lift. To compensate for this, you should take a double hop on each leg with the opposite lifting leg coming up in 2 moves. You'll find the extra time you get by hopping twice on one leg with two rotations of the rope, gives you sufficient time for a good high lift of the knee. You couldn't sustain this for 3 minutes, but you want to put in, say, 1 minute of high knee lifts every 3 minutes in a skipping routine.

There are many variations on skipping and, as with any sport, you can vary the influencing factors, the 3 principle ones being time, speed, intensity. Time is an obvious factor and speed we control by the rate of rotation of the rope. The faster we swing the rope, the quicker all our movements have to be with the legs. Intensity as the third factor can be increased over and above speed, by adding to the degree of difficulty of what we do eg. single legs, high knee lifts, weights etc etc.

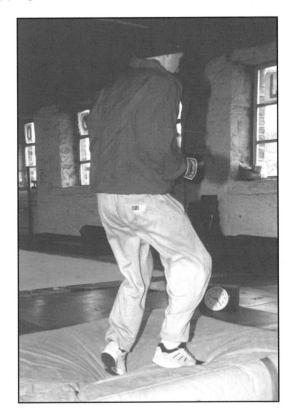

Crash Mat Jogging

If you can get onto a crash mat, then jogging on the spot with a high knee lift is a hard exercise. High hands and high knees are the order of the day and as you can see in the photograph, you need a large clock to keep track of the time - if all you're using is low technology that is!

Press Ups

For me press ups are my main 'standby' strength exercise when I'm away and unable to get into a gym. I don't do them when I can get in the gym as I've got all the equipment I need for the muscular effect.

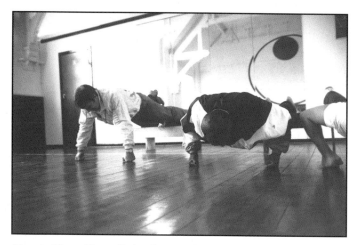

Press Ups. *Feet off the floor and onto the bench, or anything similar, so as to put more weight onto the arms. The knuckles are optional.*

In nearly all cases when I'm away I'll hit press ups twice a day. I'm not an early morning trainer, but if the day ahead looks particularly bad I'll fit in a mandatory 100 press ups and the same in Sit ups before the shower. I do them in blocks of 25ish. On the first set I could do more, but know that the second and subsequent will, as a consequence, be in the low teens which is always somewhat demoralising.

The routine is to intersperse each set with the set of sit ups. Also I vary the press up by pressing very wide to hit the shoulders and back, narrow to hit the triceps and chest more. On some sets (not too many) I'll put my thumbs together so as to drastically increase the strain on the triceps. Each day I'll also vary the routine, sometimes doing inclines, again with a narrow grip to hit the pecs., and if I can 'arrange' the furniture I will do 'dip presses' which is to have my toes on the end of the bed and my hands on the edge of two chairs which I'll 'dip' below. The form must be maintained with a perfectly straight back as always. The few inches of extra stretch seem to add pounds to your bodyweight and reps fall drastically. I can't get 25 in a set and the 'pump' is fantastic.

Press ups hit far more muscles in the body than other equipment based chest exercises would. By keeping good form you exercise both the stomach and lower back muscles. Leg muscles also come into play as the also help maintain rigidity.

Sit Ups

Like the press ups I'll vary the type of sit up that I do. Also, as with the press up, I don't rush through them, but keep the movements slow, controlled and strict. Sit ups should be done so as to ensure, apart from everything else that we hit the 'internal obliques'. These are the muscles which support the lower back. The problem is that the lower abs are not properly worked with most sit up exercises, but rather with knee raises. For this purpose, 'hanging leg raises' both to the front and to the sides are excellent .

Good form is essential and it benefits us not if we wrap our hands around our neck and then throw ourselves upwards. Fingers should touch the ears or be folded across the chest and, to make things harder, keep the elbows well back. This stops you 'rocking' them forward and if kept back increases the weight you are having to pull up. The three main muscles in the stomach are the rectus abdominus and the internal and external

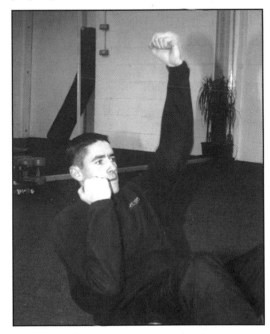

If you can lock your feet, then abdominal crunches combined with punches, as described in Chapter 8, are excellent.

obliques. As a by-product of working our 'abs' we also work the Iliacus and psoas muscles as well as the rectus femoris a major muscle in the hip joint

Unless I'm doing crunches, where I bring my shoulders off the floor and crunch up to my chest with my legs ('Scissors Crunches),I always want to lock my feet under something, such as the hotel bed. By doing this I'm able to include sets of 'rotational punches' (see the chapter on partner drills), but more importantly I'm able to properly work my obliques, both Internal and External. Crunches work the right external obliques if you move your right elbow to your left knee, but it also works your 'left Internal' at the same time - marvellous!.

Strictly for the external obliques I'll do side crunches. Cross the ankles over and get both feet locked under something. Put the hand on the floor side onto your head, just touching, with the other touching the chest. You are on your side and now crunch up about 12 inches. The rep range is only ever, for me, about 15, but it really bites into the sides.

In the early phase of a sit up, as our shoulder comes off the floor, we engage our rectus abdominus. People sometimes decry some types of sit ups as the only

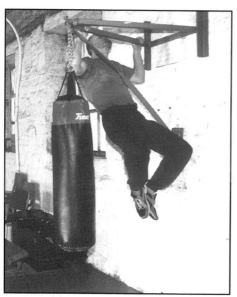

engage the Illiapsoas muscle combinations in the top of the leg, but I'm less concerned with this. Don't, however, do sit ups on the flat of your back on a flat floor - it will strain your back, as will straight leg raises fro that position. Always do sit ups and any ab work with your legs bent.

Chins

The main back strengthening exercise. In the gym I'll often fight shy of putting in the chins I know I should do, resorting to other equipment and other less demanding exercises. Chins are like squats, basic and essential. If I can't get in the gym, however, they are harder to improvise than either press ups or situps. That having been said I've chinned up the edge of a door before now using my bag gloves or socks to cushion the sharp edges. If your fingers are strong enough, you can chin off the door surround (in my case for approx 2 reps), but if you are prepared to be ingenious you can usually find somewhere to chin.

Bag Work

I can 'play' with a punch bag for ages and not get bored. Over many years, bag work has become something of a security blanket. I don't need anyone else, yet I have an opponent and I can simply 'play' by keeping the work light and fluid, both with kicks and punches or I can dig in and go for big power shots with hands and feet.

It's the latter we're going to cover here. Given this and on a personal front, I need the heavy bag and a long bag. Six foot plus and heavy is ideal. I don't want to keep chasing a light bag all over the gym and want to know that I've had to hit it with telling shots to make it move.

If you're going to do a session of bag work, then decide on a goal before you start. This might be say, 6 x 2-3 minute rounds and pre-determine the nature of the rounds. By that I mean how you pace your effort. It would be practically impossible to go completely full out for 3 minutes or, possibly even 2, but within your round you must have some peaks, which could be as long as a minute or 45 seconds. If you're going to do 6 rounds of say, 2.5 minutes, the rounds may go like this:-

Round 1 - warm up round - hands only and an easy pace, then stretch out during the 30 seconds rest, having ensured that you pre-stretched your legs and generally warmed up before you came to the bag.

Round 2 - warm up round with hands and feet. Then stretch out during the 30 seconds break.

Round 3 - hands only at a fast pace and heavier - timed so that the last 30 seconds is completely all out and as fast and as heavy as possible - rest 30 seconds

Round 4 - same as 3 but just legs, with the final 30 seconds blast - rest.

Round 5 - Hands and feet, but the emphasis is on impact. Every shot is as hard as you can make it, with big, heavy kicks and deep, penetrative punches. You have to move the bag and make it bend, however heavy it is - rest 45 seconds - 1 minute.

Round 6 - this is the all out round, where from the off, its fast and hard, with a high punch and kick rate. You will probably have to shorten the round from 2.5 minutes to 2, or from 3 minutes to 2.5, but sustain the power and speed for the whole round.

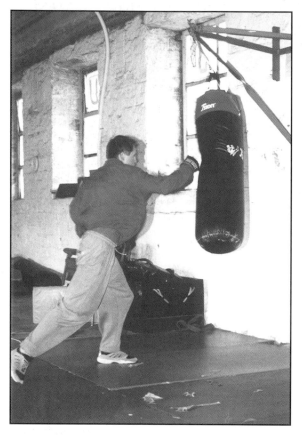

Round 5 - big, heavy shots that move the bag like this.

I'm not saying that you have to stop there on the bag after completion of the 6 rounds, as you may want to just play and practice technique for a while, but make the physical power and aggressive side of bag work, a set routine in itself.

Alternate A

If I'm on my own, I'll sometimes intersperse the bag rounds with skipping. Combining the two really hits the shoulders, upper back and arms and builds good muscle stamina. Go straight off the bag onto the skipping and vice versa. At first, when you come off the bag, skip easy, with a low leg lift until you have recovered somewhat and then vary the intensity, as your stamina allows.

You can increase the degree of difficulty of the skipping with the use of hand weights or wrist weights - see photos. Again, these will really help the skipping hit the deltoids, as you work to control the weight on the swing of the rope.

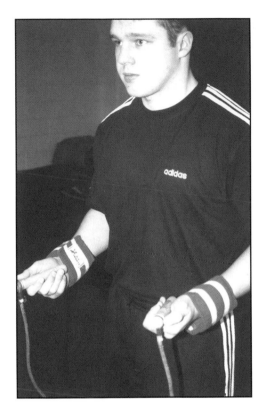

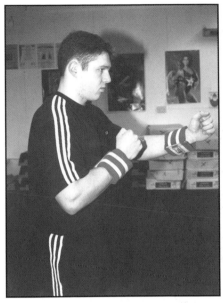

By adding velcro-fastening wristweights to skipping, alternated with Wing Chun punches and bag work, the level of intensity and improvement in muscle endurance doubles.

Alternate B

I may also add in a third exercise to this bag and skipping sequence by including some tight, fast 'Wing Chun' punches. These are illustrated in the photographs and I'll do them in combinations of 3 or 5 for no set period, simply until the lactic acid build-up stops me. To add to the degree of difficulty, I'll do these punches with the hand weights or keep the wrist weights on and by punching with this additional weight, you will very quickly reach muscle fatigue in the delts, traps, triceps and rear shoulder muscles.

Back onto the bag, initially nice and easy to shake the shoulders out and then build up the pace, making it as fast or heavy as you decide. If your goal is a specific shoulder workout, then you will want to include the close punching repetitions on the bag. These should be sustained for 30 seconds and again, punish the delts and top of the lats. The arms are held close and the elbows snapped into the punch, assisted by a little bounce of the body. You should put each punch on the same spot with both hands and keep a fast pace with a sharp snap. If you can sustain the 30 seconds with everything else that you've been doing, that's good and at completion of the time target, break off and then work normally on the bag again.

Finish the round and then back onto the skipping. You don't need to do skipping, and could include any of the 'circuit' exercises - press-ups, sit-ups, squat thrusts, star jumps etc etc. I'm all for keeping it simple, however, and am also a creature of habit. Once into a particular routine, I must admit I try and stick to it.

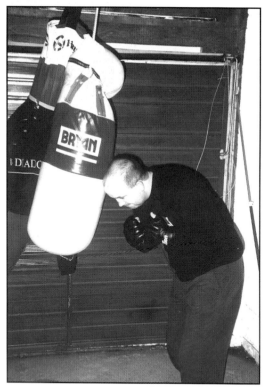

The bag can be used for every technique. Here - Geoff T. is working his 'head'. (Probably the only time he ever does - some would submit, but not this author of course!)

I don't want to go into specific techniques in this book for working the bag. I use a bag for all my visualisation work and pre-emptive strike practice - see **'Powerstrike'** and **x**. Here we are concerned about the physical effort required to complete the session, the power generated in doing so and the aggression which is needed to complete the drills and which is filed away in the sub-conscious. Like the body shield, the punch bag is unequalled in bringing out aggression.

I've always found it hard when shadow boxing or kicking, either with the benefit of a mirror or not, to feed much aggression into the technique. It seems to be a product of actually hitting something that does generate that correct feeling. At times however - particularly in the absence of any equipment, shadow boxing and kicking may be all you have.

Whilst training in Algeria this year, I included sprint shuttles on the basketball court, with kicks at the end, into the mesh fence. Whilst it became physically demanding, I just couldn't feed the aggression through into the technique and essentially, just went through the motions. Also, I have to admit that 0515 in the morning is not the time that I'm at my most aggressive, but be that as it may, I know that the ability and feeling of being able to drive blows and kicks into a heavy bag, brings out naturally a good flow of aggression.

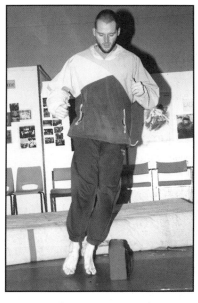

If you're on your own - ankle jumps don't need to be done over ankles - improvise.

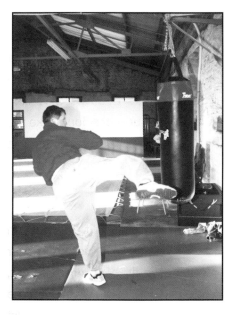

If you can't find a gym with a bag, hopefully you'll be able to buy one (the bag that is - not the gym) and get it up somewhere at home. It's the invaluable training aid and partner. It's never ill, never complains, it's always on time and above all, the bugger doesn't hit back - get one!

A heavy bag is essential for kicking.

CHAPTER 8

PARTNER DRILLS

Partner Drills

This chapter could equally be headed 'Group Drills' or even 'Individual Drills', as they can all be adapted to a group session or even modified for one person, when training on his or her own.

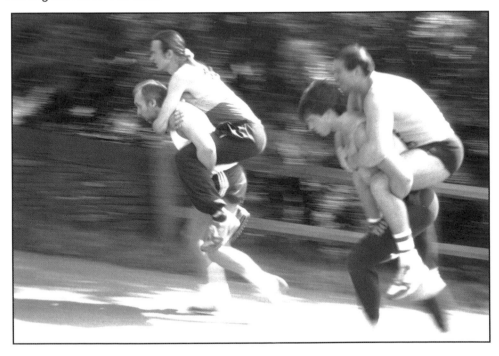

Hill Carries - certainly fall under the heading of 'Stress Drills'. If there are enough of you, then any competitive element in an exercise such as this is good.

Partner training has innumerable advantages. Many training routines can be doubled by the presence of a partner, such as hill work routines. A partner or partners gives a competitive edge and commits us at all times to give everything to the drills and the session. I also accept that all the drills we covered on the chapter headed 'Equipment', was with a partner, but I've separated the two, as those are essentially performed without the use of combative equipment. Most of the drills we're going to look at fall under the following heading do not use equipment. They may, however, be done inside or outside as occasion and circumstances demand.

Stress Drills

This sub-title also seems somewhat inappropriate, as all the drills in this book are performed under the general principle that stress is an inherent factor, but I've given this title specifically to the following drills as they are introductory drills, with which you can start a session and which wake everyone up. After a warm-up and then a stretch out, you can throw in a combination of these drills. They are exacting, hit the lungs immediately and also challenge aerobic capacity.

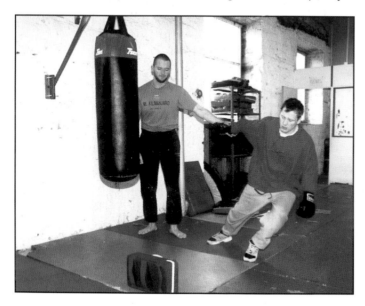

Wind Sprints - a good push off and a good low turn. Your partner must keep a keen eye on the clock. In this case it's behind the pad.

Drill 1 - Wind Sprints

Your partner paces out a good 12 metres and then sets himself with a firm upright stance, with one arm held rigid in front. On a timed signal, you sprint to him and can push off his hand to help you turn, sprint back and touch the start point with your foot, or the bottom of a wall, if you're in a gym and then sprint back.

The sprinting continues for 30 seconds. There is a 15 second break and a second sprint for 30 seconds by the same person. At the end of this set you should feel as if you can't do anymore - unfortunately, you've got just 15 seconds to get yourself mentally prepared for the last set of a further 30 seconds of sprints and you should be 'hanging out' by the time you've finished.

If you've put everything into the first 2 sets, you should feel as if you don't have it in you physically for the last set and that's how it should be. This is the feeling we're trying to duplicate, so that only strong mental resolve and focus will enable you to finish. As an aid, your partner counts the number of runs you made on each 30 second sprint ie. 12 - 11 - 11 or 10 - 11 - 8.

Surprisingly, there is usually a good start, a less successful second sprint, yet the last, can often equal the first if the mental attitude is right. However, a lesser number on the second set can often indicate that this particular sprint has been 'paced'. Count only those shuttles, that when the stop signal comes, places the man over the imaginary halfway line from his start point to his partner. Change partners and repeat the dose as required.

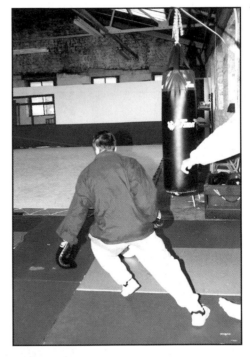

A powerful push-off in the turn is what wind sprints are all about. This puts a heavy load on the lower quads and builds power.

Technical Tip

Keep low on the turns and lean back into the direction you'll be going when you turn. Power out of the turn so that you really use your leg muscles to accelerate. Stopping at the end of the sprint, before the turn, also takes a degree of muscular effort and it's definitely a drill for the shorter, more powerful sprinter to whom turning is less of an effort.

Make sure, as the static partner, that you provide a firm arm to push off on the turn, give a good warning of the time, particularly during the 15 seconds break. Hurry your partner back to his start line and give him a countdown ie. "5 seconds to go - get ready". Also, get him in the right aggressive frame of mind.

I used to do wind sprints on my own 20 odd years ago, across the width of a sprint track. I used to time myself and despite the degree of difficulty in pushing oneself, it is possible to 'work the watch' and sprint. I've used car parks, deserted roads - running from kerb edge to kerb edge and anywhere that will fit the bill. You can put wind sprints in at the end of your 30 minutes run - say 2-3 sets or combine them with high knee lifts - see below.

Drill 2 - High Knee Lifts

As with wind sprints, a one or two man drill. This is an old sprint training exercise, for me is one of the best drills for building leg strength, particularly lifting strength in the upper thighs and illiapsoas muscles and also developing determination.

When with a partner, as in Drill 1, 10-12 metres is a good distance. With one person facing his partner, he sets off with the exercise. Whilst the same distance in the wind sprint would be covered in about 3 seconds or less, high knee lifts take over 15 - 20 seconds and there should be some 40 - 50 steps made in the process. As you pass your partner, he sets off back to your start point and this is your recovery period. As he passes the point at which you started, you set off again towards him and he gets himself ready and tries to recover, ready for you to get to

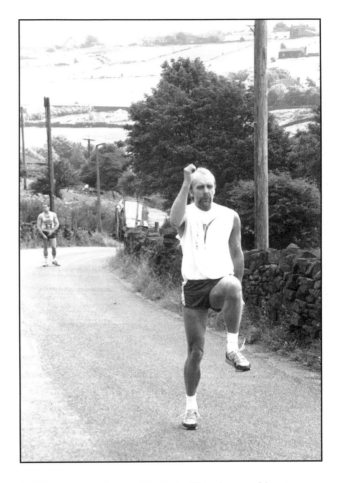

High Knee Lifts on the hill. *This time working to a set distance - one man goes, then the next. This way you can work your way up a long hill in stages.*

him so that he can then set off again - and so on.

Depending on fitness levels, you will want to put in at least 4 shuttles each and probably no more than 6.

Technical Tip

High knee lifts, unfortunately, demand a bit more application of technique than the other drills in this section. The first point is that you must lean back - if you don't, you will restrict the rise of your knees. To help in this, look up to the sky, forget the finish line and kick your knees high up into your chest. Take short, stabbing strides, covering little ground and where you take 20 seconds to cover the same distance as you sprinted in 3, you end up with 40 - 50 strides instead of 8 - 10.

The arms are of considerable importance in the high knee lift and this is where some problems of co-ordination can arise, particularly for those people new to it. You must develop a big arm swing, high up to the sky, which helps throw your bodyweight upwards each time. This helps 'buy the time' for your knees to be high in the air and the whole thing should co-ordinate nicely - some chance! I've seen people perform like pregnant dodos the first time they try it, but eventually achieve some degree of technique.

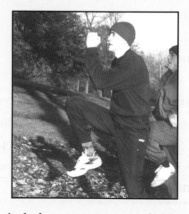

Your partner is there to encourage and particularly to ensure you maintain the high knee action and don't incline to taking too long a stride. This is where, performing on your own is difficult. The main problem is timing rest periods. I've always had a problem in getting the right balance on the rest period and, consequently, when doing them on my own, prefer to put them into hill work. The rest period is then simply the recovery whilst walking back down to the start line. The distance should be the same but don't pick too steep a hill to do high knee lifts on - it's an exacting enough exercise as it is without overdoing it.

DRILL 3 - ANKLE JUMPS

These should be done after the wind sprints or high knee lifts. They are used as a 'finishing' exercise after something which has been more demanding and draining.

As the photographs show, one person lies down and puts their feet together. On the signal, the partner will hop, from side to side, with one bounce on each side of the ankle for 30 seconds. The break is 15 seconds and then off again. The repeats can be for two more sets of 30 seconds, but, if you're doing them after something else, you might make the sequence 30 seconds and 15 seconds rest - 20 seconds and 10 seconds rest and 15/20 seconds on the final push.

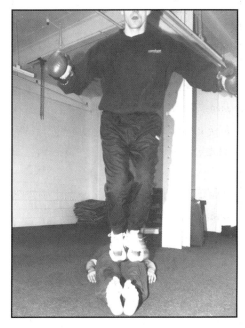

You must maintain the rhythm and the main work is taken on the calves and lower thighs and knee support muscles. Make sure you bounce back on each bounce - not as some people do, which is stop and then push off again. A 30 second set, should see some 50 springs over the ankles and your partner should count how many and let you know.

Technical Tip

Spring your feet up to a reasonable height and use your hands as 'counter weights' to help turn your body slightly from side to side, so that on each bounce you are facing the way you're next going to spring. If you notice from the photographs, the head tends to remain vertical, over the same spot, with the body, when it hits the ground, being at an angle. It is this that demands you immediately spring back, otherwise you would fall over. Where people go wrong is that they spring their body vertically over the ankles and fail to achieve the necessary demand to spring back before falling. With some practice, you'll get it so that you won't miss a beat. It's a lot like skipping and you will need to master the co-ordination, so as to get the best out of it physically.

Drill 3A - Bench Jumps

A variation of ankle jumps, bench jumps are ideal for single or group work. As the photos show you can use a proper bench if you can find one, or you can

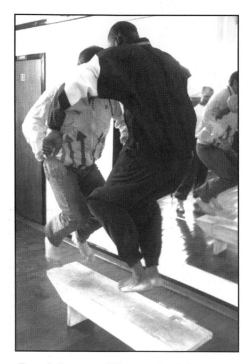

compromise with whatever you can find. The way to do them is to try and keep the head at the same height and mount the bench by bending at the knees. As with all 'springing' exercises it's important that you come straight back off the floor

You can also use a chair by stepping on and off it for 30 secs, say, or as long as you feel. The important thing is if you use a chair that you keep on one leg for half of the time allotted and then change legs. With a chair you are not springing up, rather stepping up, but if done properly it can be taxing. When you use a chair you must make sure that you stand up all the way and straighten your legs - don't shorten

Bench Jumps - *Where timing is important, as you both need to co-ordinate - or else.*

the step up so that you just touch the chair edge and come back down.

Drill 4 - Down - Stretch - Sprint

A drill for 4 or more people and one where good teamwork is essential if everyone is to get something out of it.

Start off standing and on the command ***'Down',*** drop into a lying position and on the second command ***'Stretch',*** make sure your arms are pushed forward and your legs pushed out behind. Following a slight hold, the third command is ***'Sprint'.*** Use the arms to pull and push up and the legs to power away into the sprint. At the pre-determined 10 - 12 metre line, the command 'Down' is given, followed by 'Stretch' and then 'Sprint'. If there are, say, 5 people in the line, then each person gives 4 sprint commands and then passes control to the next one in the line.

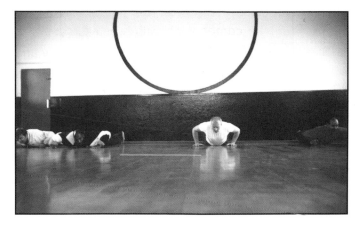

Above and to the right - **Down** *and* **Stretch.** *Whoever is calling can hold marginally on the stretch to ensure that everyone complies.*

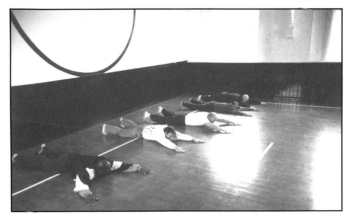

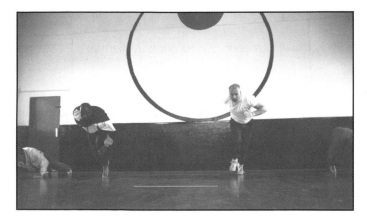

Some readers might uncharitably think that your much loved author took a flyer on the **Sprint** *command. (You'd be right, but I didn't fool my partner on my right - damn!).*

Each person has the ability to control the pace, sometimes holding on the stretch until a slower member has caught up, or to force any people who are guilty, to emphasise the 'Stretch' and not just pay lip service with a short reach forward. With 5 people, you have 20 sprints, which is exhausting. One set of these is really enough. As with the last drill, a certain 'experience of technique', eventually helps, but even the most untrained will get a heavy push from it.

Technical Tip

Don't ignore the arms and use them for pulling yourself forward off the ground, which is why the 'Stretch' portion is emphasised. Keep low as you come off the ground into the sprint and on the turn, endeavour to make the turn whilst stopping, so that you are throwing yourself to the ground whilst still on the move. If you master a good start and a fast turn, you'll just buy those extra few seconds which may make a difference in your pace compared to others.

A very important aspect is to count the sprints. Don't let others down by not being aware that the person next to you has finished his own count. A smooth transition of control down the line makes for the best physical returns for everyone.

Drill 5 - Sprints on the Spot

When there are a few people, accelerated sprints on the spot are best done in a circle. This way nobody can cheat. Start off with a jog on the spot. Lean over slightly, whilst you keep on your toes and pump your legs up and down. One person has a watch and acts as timekeeper and gives the command 'Sprint'. At that, everyone sprints on the spot, as fast as his or her legs will go with no let up and with power - it can be sustained for any period you want, but somewhere between 15 - 30 seconds is very adequate. The command 'Jog' is given and this rest period, again can be between 15 - 30 seconds and then the sprint starts again. Rest and repeat the dose as required. There should be a minimum of 4 sprints, that is somewhere between 1 and 2 minutes of spaced, but fast and hard sprints on the spot.

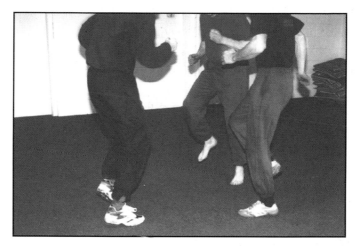

Sprinting on the spot - *if done properly can be a really demanding drill. You should put it in between an exercise which is lower leg based ie. wind sprints or even skipping.*

Technical Tip

The arms don't do anything - keep them in a high guard position and they'll naturally act as counter-weights. Also try and get a good knee lift, although its pretty much impossible if you really go fast, which is the main goal, but try to reach a compromise. Lean over and look at your feet. Fitness depending, you may want to start off just putting in 10 - 15 second sprints.

Drill 6

Another drill based on jogging on the spot and is very similar to a 'circuit training' exercise. It's best done with a small group, where 2 or 3 work whilst 2 or 3 rest and control the action.

Start jogging on the spot until you get a command to perform a set of exercises. This could be any one of the following:- Press-Ups, Squat Thrusts (feet together or alternate leg thrusts), Crunches, Star Jumps or Squat Thrust into a Star Jump. Whichever exercise is given, it should be no longer than 10 - 12 reps, but they should be done with perfect style and no cheating.

A variation on this is to give some punching and kicking commands after the technique on the ground eg. after the press-ups, people come up into a fighting stance and on command throw a combination of left jab to the face and reverse punch to the stomach. This could be repeated 6 or 8 times and with tired arms, requires a big effort.

Similarly, after the squat thrusts you would do kicks, as the legs are pumped. If you don't do any punching or kicking within the drill, then keep the jogging interval short - in other words - keep the recovery time short.

Technical Tip

The object with all these drills is the pressure to start a particular exercise, or new set at a time when you don't feel ready, that is, perfectly recovered. You are pushed to go when you are still distressed from the last set, but you have no choice - go you must. This duplicates the fight scenario, where you are probably never really mentally ready to fight, very easily tire and very quickly feel like giving up. These exercises, at the risk of repeating myself ad nauseum, condition your sub-conscious into knowing that however bad you feel physically, that you can actually 'go again' and achieve a good result.

Drill 7 - Incline Ab Punches

One of the hardest drills for the abs, particularly the obliques - both internal and external. We use this normally as a partner drill but you can do them on your own if you can 'lock' your feet. Remember - always keep your knees bent.

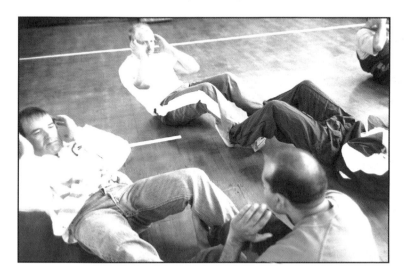

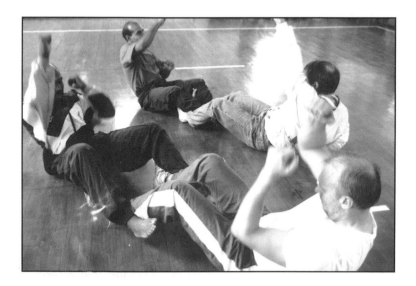

Slow abdominal crunches and inclined punching. One of the hardest exercises for the abs there is - particularly the external and internal obliques.

Start the exercise with 15 very slow crunches, working from the 'small' of your back only touching the floor, not the shoulders. Come up to an upright position but do not rest at the top. Try to keep continuous tension on the stomach and by keeping this phase slow, nobody can throw themselves up. Keep the tips of your fingers touching your ears, again so that no assistance can be gained from pulling up. The important point here is to try to keep the elbows back, which places more weight behind you.

After the 15 slow reps, lean back to an angle of 30 degrees. Raise a punching arm vertically above the head and put the other arm by your side. You're now going to perform repetition of punches, just as you would if you were lined up in a martial arts class ie. one punch after the other. Twist the trunk on each punch at a reasonable pace for 40 punches. Don't, however, punch too fast just to get it over with quickly. Make sure you twist into each punch and pull back simultaneously and strongly with the other hand to help this.

When you've finished the 40 punches, this is the end of the first set and rest for 15-20 seconds and start the second set. This time reduce the sit-ups to 12 reps and increase the punches to 60. Rest - now 10 sit-ups and 80 punches.
Rest - and finally 8 very slow sit-ups and 100 punches. If you can complete this properly the first time, you can throw this book away - you don't need it. Very few people, even those with strong abs can do the last set without a break. If you need to build up to it, adjust the number of sit-ups and punches to suit.

Technical Tip

Always monitor yourself and others to ensure that when punching, they are leaning back at a low angle of 30 degrees and not at 45 or more, which takes considerable strain off the stomach. Also ensure that people punch directly above their heads and not punching forward. This ensures you keep the weight of your arms high above you and not in front. To ensure this happens, people can look up, although I find that this can often cause a strain on the neck, so allow people to look forward but make sure they realise where they are punching.

Hill Carries

The 'Hill Work' described in Chapter 7 work equally as well for partner training, in fact the potential range of exercises are increased as well as variations on a theme and one of these, is the hill carry.

With 2 or more people you have many variations to work on. The main addition to be made is the 'hill carry'. I found it one of the most testing of training routines over the years and the one most people avoid.The way I work it is the same way I've always done.

The Drill

One person 'mounts up' and sets off up a short and reasonably steep slope. At the top both come down and the person who was carrying lines up in front of his partner. This has all been without any delay and on a command from

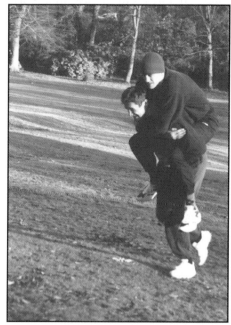

Hill Carry - note the good, high carry position and the hands locked to take the strain off the biceps.

his partner he sprints back up the hill with his partner in pursuit shouting words of encouragement or some such thing.

Both back down and now the first person gets a rest while he is carried up the hill, until its his turn to go again, after sprinting behind his partner. Change again and so on. After 4 sets each of the carry and sprints you'll have had enough. Don't be too ambitious at first, remember, intensity on a hill is a combination of 3 things - the steepness of the hill, the distance you travel and lastly, the speed. You can make hill carries as varied as you want, but if the hill is steep then shorten the carry and the subsequent sprint to only 20 metres or so.

Technical Tip

The first consideration of hill carries is avoidance of injuries. The obvious potential injury is to your lower back, but this is avoided by good technique. The 'mount-up' is achieved by your partner getting a good high jump and you getting a good high carry position with him. He should sit comfortably above your hip bones and you should get a good locked position with your arms under his legs.

On the shorter carries you don't need to lock your fingers together, as the weight on your biceps is only for a short period. On the longer carries you need to lessen the strain on the arms, by either interlacing your fingers or gripping the ends of your fingers with each hand. You'll find that if you don't lock your hands on a long carry, he'll start to slip down your hips, which will both break your concentration and strain your biceps.

On a grass slope, particularly if wet, grip and foot placement is the key. Keep your strides very short. Don't reach too high with your steps and make sure you've got a good firm foot placement before you take the weight. I train in fell running shoes and always have. They are reasonably light, have a good outdoor sole which grips on wet grass and still work for road work and pad work kicking. Currently I use Merrell 'Trails', but any light fell shoe will do.

Long Hill Carry

An alternative and one that tests both anaerobic and aerobic fitness is the long carry. This involves finding a hill of say 3/4 of a mile or so with a reasonable angle. Decide on the changeover point which may be 80 or 100 or 120 strides. One person mounts up and off he goes as fast as he can. Both count the strides and the partner being carried just shouts on every 20 strides and then shouts change on the prescribed point. A quick, on the move change and your off again. With 4 or 6 people you can get a good race going. A degree of competitiveness adds stress and tension and makes it a punishing exercise. I've used it on Bodyguard training courses for many years as a means of separating the fit from the not and it's also a great feeling to finish, never mind to win.

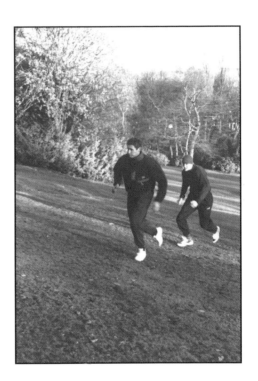

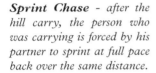

Sprint Chase - *after the hill carry, the person who was carrying is forced by his partner to sprint at full pace back over the same distance.*

Hare and Hounds (Sprinting)

This allows you to 'factor in' age and sprinting ability into your partner training. Rarely do people train together who have equal ability and fitness. Whether on the hill or the flat it is a good routine to 'stagger' the starting line up. Give the slowest person a 5 stride advantage, say, which is then the start point. The signal to go is when that person makes a move. He can, reasonably hold the start for as long as he wants and can try and catch his partner or partners off guard. It creates tension, competition and more importantly it should mean, providing the 'handicap' has been accurate, that people finish together.

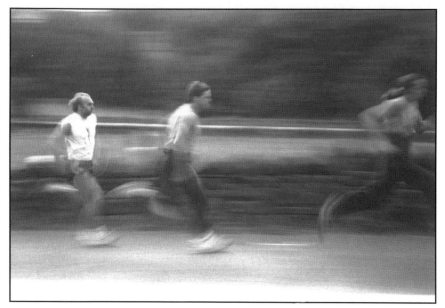

Hare and Hounds. *Those of you, who by now, may have grown fond of your author, need not worry - I'm bringing up the rear in order to create a false sense of security in my partners.*

It is demoralising, if when sprinting against someone, they pull way ahead. The incentive to push hard is lost and, equally, for the person in front he can relax if he is way ahead. A staggered sprint pushes both people, who should finish 'neck and neck'. This is the essence of partner training and improves the 'output of effort' over training on your own many fold. It works for me in all circumstances whether its on the pads, hill, or weights.

Long hill Sprint and 'Kick Sprint'

Long sprints, is an incorrect title as it's not possible to sprint any reasonable distance on a hill. More correctly this section should be titled long hill 'Push' and kick sprint, as the run actually becomes a sustained push at probably 75% of the maximum you could hit the hill at over, say, half the distance.

Find a reasonably steep hill, approx. 200m in length. With your partner, set off at what we said is a sustained push. Don't under run. It's hard to decide the necessary amount of effort, but it's a pace at which you know you have some effort and speed in reserve. The feeling is definitely unlike the 'hare and hounds' at this stage.

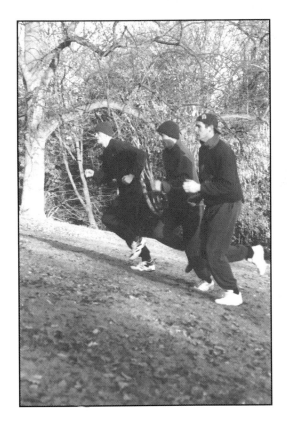

*Now the **Kick Sprint** after the long push. The tree on the right has been chosen as the marker to start the sprint for the final 50 metres or so.*

However, at a pre-determined point - fixed visually by the side of the road or track you both feed in the full sprint speed and all out effort - this is probably at the 150m mark. It's now a competitive sprint for the finish and what you're doing is training your body and mind to be capable of giving that 'extra' push, particularly when you are exhausted, because at the 150m mark you should have set a pace which was one where you have reached a physical finish point.

This is one of the most taxing drills you can do and one that takes a big mental effort. For those of you who have seen the **'Fit To Fight'** video you'll remember the opening sequence with some runners cresting a hill. They are running on the pavement in a domestic area. My old training partner for many years, Neil Rigby and myself would use that for the 'finish' of our step work - also shown on the video.

We'd use this steep hill for the long push and kick sprint session. The lamposts would be our visual reference for the sprint part and if we were doing three sets we would move the kick sprint point further up the hill by one lampost each time so as to shorten the sprint distance. Whilst the sprint distance is shorter the long 'push' is more and you are longer on the hill so putting more effort into it that way. On the last one the burn in the arse defies description, particularly given the very delicate nature of the people who are reading this book - doormen and the like!

This training gives us that 'mental switch' that we need to have in a fight so as to move up a gear at any point, however exhausted we may be. You will demoralise anyone you are up against if you can 'explode' with renewed energy.

CHAPTER 9

EQUIPMENT DRILLS

Equipment and Drills

The equipment I always want to include in my training routines are the punching and kicking shields and the hook & jab mits. Variations on a theme such as the smaller air shields, large forearm pads or heavy Thai pads are also excellent.

I am after 4 main effects from pad work:-

1. Maintenance of Technique/Timing

2. Power

3. Stamina Building & Anaerobic Capacity

4. Aggression

With pad work, unlike the weights, or running, or CV machine work, we are now much closer to the hub of the wheel. Working on pads, we are working techniques which are combative and which we may have to use. However, due to the way we work the pads and to maintain interest and mental complexity, we will probably work techniques and combinations of techniques we'll never use in the streets.

I separate how I use such equipment when I want to achieve purely impact techniques and how I work with them for fitness and mobility. In this book we'll only be looking at the drills which basically subscribe to the latter effects. The pre-supposition is that you have, of course, a partner. The piece of equipment for all this without a partner is the punchbag, but more on this later.

As with the weights, we're going to work broad groups with a wide variety of exercises and drills. My favourite piece of equipment has to be the 'Boss' instructors shield. A combination of high density polystyrene and foam inner, covered by a corfam outer, produces a training aid unequalled as far as I'm concerned. When either kicking or punching, it's demands on your anaerobic capacity and muscle endurance is terrific. This is because the energy of your technique is absorbed, there's no bounce off it or recoil or recovery that you may get from a heavy bag or more solid hook & jab mit. It soaks up every technique and drains you of energy within the first minute. It also allows your partner to 'feedback' to you how effective your shots are and it can, surprisingly, be used in a variety of ways.

Over many years, the techniques haven't changed from those I used to train with when in Manchester and Lance Lewis was in charge of a group of us who trained weekly with the shields as the basis for Full Contact. Such luminaries as Brian Seabright, Chris Williams, Chris Boughey and many others of note, joined in these sessions in those days, some foolishly more consistently than others and with the exception of the training sessions in Huddersfield with Bob and Tony Sykes, have been the hardest martial arts training I've ever done.

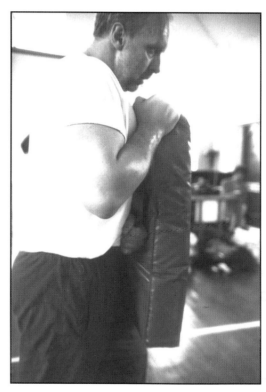

The correct hold for the **'Shield'**. *Held firmly to the body so as to give a good solid feel for the kicker or puncher.*

The benefit of such work is that it is 'use specific'. We work the body to the point of muscle and cardiovascular fatigue, but by using techniques of punching and kicking that we will need in practical terms at some time.

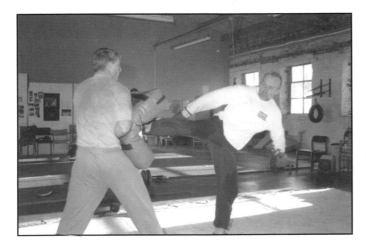

Even when working for endurance over 2 minutes - we still need to put big, power shots in, that bend the shield.

None of the techniques with the body shield are stationary. They work either on the advance, retreat, linked with shuttle runs or with complete freedom of movement. The first drills we're going to look at are 'retreats'. The benefit of these are that we learn to kick whilst on the move, going backwards and whilst of little practical value, certainly in the street, it demands and improves timing to achieve a solid hit and particularly develops good balance.

Drill 1 - Retreats - Shield

One person, we'll call him 'the opponent' edges forward at a very slow walk, advancing towards his partner. The drill is purely a kicking drill and the object is for the retreating person to work 'stop kicks'. You can restrict the kicks to only front kicks, only side kicks, only back kicks, or only jumping kicks or, on the third or fourth set, you will include all kicks and always include jumping kicks, which have the advantage of including some plyometric effort into the

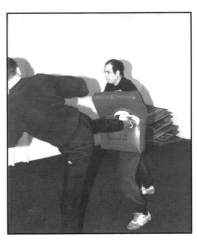

Side 'Stop Kick' - on the retreat. The shield man constantly 'edges' forward.

exercise. Those people who know my views on martial arts and self defence, know full well that I'm never going to advocate jumping kicks for the street, but they are hard to do, they are even harder to do well, even harder to do well with tired legs, even harder to do on the retreat and, in summary, nearly impossible to do well with tired legs on the retreat, whilst trying to place them accurately and with power. The result is a very testing drill, which is hard work. The jumping kicks are helping develop the 'plyometric' effect and are draining.

If you restrict the retreats to sets of specific kicks, then on the final one, you should allow all kicks and you should do 2 sets eg.

Set A - Retreat Front Kicks

Set B - Retreat Back Kicks

Set C - Retreat Side Kicks

Set D - Retreat Jumping Kicks

Set E - Retreat All Kicks

Set F - Repeat Set E

These should be done across the narrow part of a training hall, which is a pretty meaningless statement, but ideally, it should be no wider than 15 metres. You have a number of ways of doing the exercise ie. one person can do all 6 sets by turning at the end of one set and retreating back, however, it can probably be too taxing and to maintain power and technique, probably better if at the end of each set, there is a changeover of kicker.

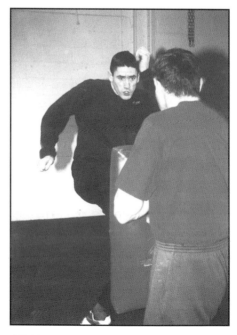

Kicking on the retreat - tests all skills, particularly balance.

Drill 2 - Shuttle Run

The next drill is the 'shuttle run'. In the bad old days when I trained this drill with Lance Lewis, we used to start these with either 10 press-ups or a rope climb in the college gym we used at that time.

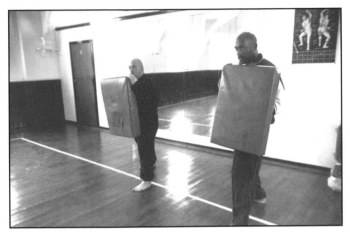

Waiting for the kickers to sprint down for the **Shuttle Runs.**

One person holds a shield in a fixed solid position, with a high stance and the pad, as always, fixed squarely against the chest and abdomen. The opponent has a 'sprint' down to the pad and then 4 - 6 kicks. Allow the whole range of kicks from front kicks, side, jumping and spinning kicks, but exclude roundhouse kicks, as the pad needs to stay facing forward. At the end of the kicks, the kicker sprints back to his start point, turns and sprints back to the shield for another 4 - 6 kicks.

This is repeated 4 - 6 times, depending on the length of the run. If you can get a longish gym, eg. 25 metres, make it 4 shuttles - if you're restricted for space make it 6. With a drill such as this, to have 4 - 6 people training is good because the element of competition, particularly with regard to sprint speed, enters into the equation. However, the downside of this is that kicks can be rushed and this isn't the object. Each kick, however tired the legs, particularly towards the end, must be delivered accurately and with full power on every occasion. Then change partners.

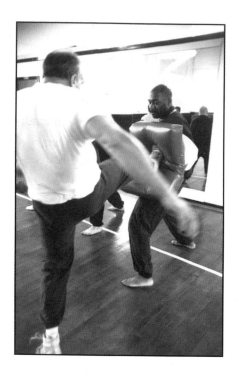
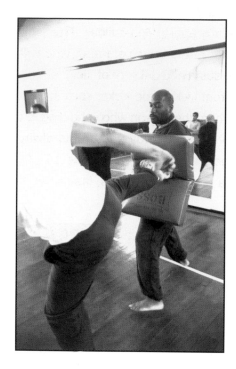

Drill 2. *Having sprinted down, the above shows 2 out of a 4 or 5 kick sequence. You could include spinning kicks, jumping kicks or kicks off the front and back legs. No roundhouse kicks.*

Below - sprinting back to the start for another shuttle run back to the pads.

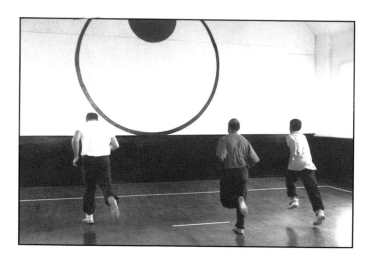

Drill 3 - Advances - Shield

A big aggression-builder. This is the advance, and on this occasion, opposite to drill 1, it is the shield man who will retreat. At the signal, the kicker attacks with a sustained delivery of kicks of all descriptions, apart from roundhouse type kicks. Front kicks, side kicks, spinning back kicks, knees even, are blasted into the pad, where the person who is holding it, allows himself to be kicked back at a measured, even and steady pace. This always keeps the kicker within a good distance of the shield. It may only take 15 - 20 seconds to complete the set, but it is with a barrage of continuous, fast, powerful kicks.

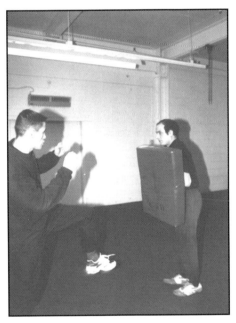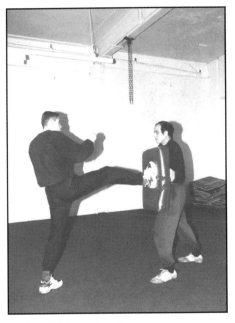

Left - a good guard, with the knee 'chambered' for a front kick on the advance.
Right - Piling in the kick on the advance, with the intention to kick your opponent backwards and then to advance into the next kick.

Its a complete release of aggression and you can generate tremendous power and impact as your momentum builds. Accuracy, precision, technique and balance are all fundamentals for any kicking exercise and these should not be sacrificed in the interest of throwing oneself at the shield. Try and finish with a really big powerful kick to blast your partner back on the last shot. Change over and restrict this drill to only 2 each. On a safety point, the shield man must be careful that with any retreat he does with a shield, that this is only after the kick is landed and not during it's delivery. The obvious dangers to the knee joint need no amplification and as with all pad work, there is as much skill and timing in holding the pads, or shield in this case, as kicking or punching them.

Drill 4 - Shield Rounds

This is the culmination of the previous kicking work on the shield. For me, there isn't anything to compare, for building anaerobic tolerance, power and aggression, as there is when performing rounds on the pads.

Again, it's broken down into 4 broad divisions - front kicks - including jumping kicks, side kicks, again with jumps if you wish, back kicks to include jumping, spinning kicks and now, roundhouse kicks. Unlike the other exercises, the man holding the shield now has complete control and responsibility as to whether the session works or not. Hold the shield tight to the body, square on as previously detailed and be prepared to take and absorb the impact.

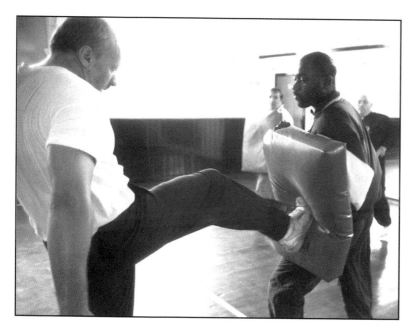

Shield Rounds.
2 minutes, all out with front kicks. Make sure you bend that shield on each kick.

There are 2 ways to do this drill:-

1. Make the man stay on the shield for the whole session or alternate after each set. If you keep one man on the shield for all the sets, the level fitness has to be exceptional, otherwise, you will have too long a session for one person to adequately maintain a high level of performance on each set. Allow no more than 30 seconds rest if you adopt this particular choice.

2. The better approach is simply to swap over after each set and get your 2 minutes rest - after a fashion - whilst holding the shield. I'm personally more in favour of this approach, as each person is better prepared for the next round. We've done it the other way but quality and power soon fall off.

First, front kicks. The man holding the shield makes his opponent kick on the retreat and on the advance, turns him and issues necessary commands if he sees that there is favouritism towards using a 'preferred' leg. He'll raise the shield a few inches to indicate that a jumping kick is required and encourage more power by asking his opponent to kick harder. He'll also watch for poor technique and ensure, above everything, that two things happen.

The first is that the kicker keeps up a good 'kick rate', as pacing the time on the shield is not what it's about. If you're doing 1.5 minutes or the full 2 minute round, then there should be a good kick rate. Also, kicks should be in combinations as well as single big power kicks. The second important aspect the shield man controls is the knee height of the kicker. The knee lift is one of the single

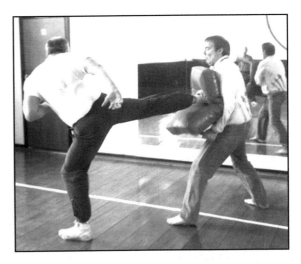

2 minutes of side kicks and make the person holding the pad 'wince'. You must try to knock him out with the power of the kick through the pad.

most important parts of the front kick. Power from the kick should travel through the shield in a straight line, horizontal to the floor - this means a good high knee lift to 'chamber' the leg.

After 1 minute on the shield, keeping the knee high on each kick is the single most difficult thing to do and this is what the shield work is all about. It is important that the shield man, whilst staying mobile, never pulls himself too far away from the kicker, which allows a breathing space.

After the 4 alternating rounds of individual kicks, it's 2 minutes of all kicks - all out. By this stage, the muscles are gone and the stamina is failing and it's here that the aggression and, to a lesser extent, technique take over. If you've out everything into the earlier rounds, then you're at the state we want to achieve in training, which is that you will get to the end of the 2 minutes as a result of one thing and one thing only - mental attitude. This is what FIT TO FIGHT is all about. This is what separates training for fitness and technique and training for a far greater effect. The mental strength these drills create and the aggression through application of power, don't desert a person as do physical strength or fitness. The mental effect and benefit of hard training is a more or less permanent feature - you know you've got it and it's there when you need it.

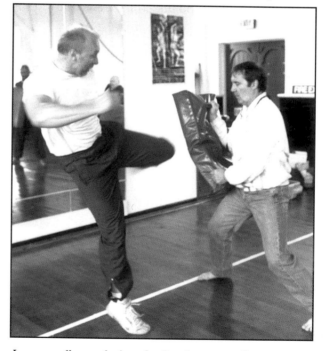

Low roundhouse during the 2 minute roundhouse session. Kicks should be high and low, left and right and you can also on this drill include high spinning kicks. As with the kick above, all out power even at 1min 59secs.

How you feel after that first minute of the last round is how you feel after 10 or 15 seconds of a fight - out of breath, weak, exhausted, failing, hollow and empty and powerless - but you have another minute to go.

Drill 5 - Body Shield - Punching
The shield is ideal for punching. It works because the pad man can give signals to vary the types of attack. There are many variations of punching that you can duplicate with the shield, which is really everything you can do on a bag and more, but with the added advantage of more mobility and feedback as to the degree of impact, which a bag does not give.

What's lost is speed ie. the speed of moving from hooks to say, uppercuts, which could happen on hook & jab mits, but the shield's main purpose is not to duplicate that fast action. The purpose of the shield is to build and develop big power shots, test aerobic capacity and anaerobic tolerance and aggression.

Rounds can be 1 minute, through to a maximum of 2 minutes. If you can go longer, you need to increase the 'dig' you're putting into the technique. You should be trying to dig right through the pad and into the man, just as you did with the kicks. The object is not to perform fast, snapping punches, which only have a surface impact. This is where the power of techniques comes into play and this is where base strength is often not the answer.

Whilst we are not after fast, snapping shots, we still want fast punches, without sacrificing power and a good punch rate ie. keep the number of punches up within any round - don't take breathers. Keep close to the shield and if you're the man holding the shield, work your man by making him follow your circling moves, retreats, punching on the advance into him and then standing your ground whilst you change the signals from the pad. I've seen fit men wilt after 1.5 minutes and be sick at the end of 2.

The shield soaks up all the impact you give it and demands that you apply every ounce of technique and dynamics in attaining powerful blows. What you don't get is 'recoil' as you would off a heavy punchbag. With all these drills on shields, pads, hook & jab mits, it's still important that your framework of technique is good. Don't get sloppy, endeavour to maintain a guard - which is a very personal thing and keep good mobility and balance.

Drill 6 - Hook & Jab

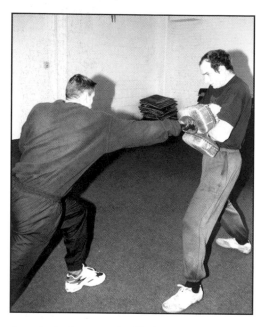

Low, body shot onto the Thai pads, during a 2-minute session.

This is one of the most exacting training drills when done correctly. The preserve, historically, of boxing training. The hook & jab mits, or focus mits, as you'll hear them referred to, have now been hijacked by martial artists. Anyone who puts on a pair of bag gloves and works out with a partner, should include this work in their training. One impediment to this is that often people are uncomfortable in holding the pads, as they feel they are looking inept.

Done badly, they do look like crap, but don't let that detract from the training benefit in using them. We're not trying to be boxers, but if we can achieve half the fitness of a good amateur or average pro boxer, then we'll be fit to fight. If use of the hook & jab mits, however amateurishly done, can achieve this, then all well and good. This doesn't mean that you shouldn't endeavour to improve your technique and range of combinations in holding the pads and if you have the bottle, take yourself off to a boxing gym or, as a secondary solution, take yourself off to a good 'boxercise' class.

The mits are to work combinations and to work them at speed. The speed of the hand combination is what now creates the physical demand, plus accuracy and body mobility. What also taxes muscle stamina is the 'recovery' of the hands from each technique, as there is little recoil from the pads. Impact on the mits is achieved by a totally different technique than that you would need when attempting to get impact on the body shield. If you try big, power shots on the mits, you'll achieve very little. Fast, snapping punches - quickly recovered, are the order of the day. The mit man exercises complete control on pace and nature of the work carried out.

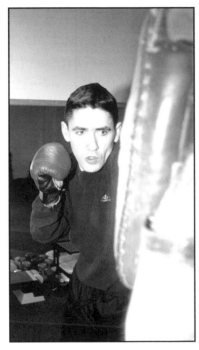

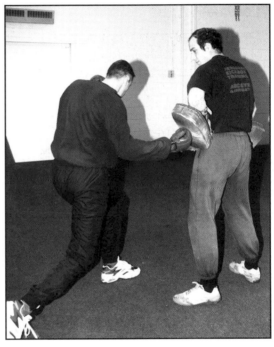

Pierre Mahon - Thai Boxer
Always keep a good guard, when working on the pads.

A low body shot onto the pad - this would naturally be followed by a left hook or a high left roundhouse.

If you can kick and have these skills, then incorporate kicking into work with the hook & jab mits. Often though, the kicking becomes very 'flicky' and given the light weight build of most boxing mits, it may be better to resort to the use of the larger padded rectangular forearm shields or heavy Thai pads, when you want to combine hands and feet. These do not drain you in anything like the same way as the shields, as their firmness will help 'recoil' the leg and hand. Impact is not absorbed in the same way as the shield and because of that, they are kinder on technique, but that for what we are after, is of lesser importance.

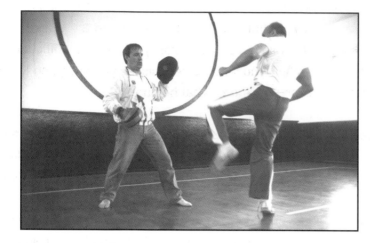

Unlike boxers, we add kicks into the Hook & Jab work.
Ged Moran - *5th Dan Karate - holding.*

Drill 7 - Pad Pyramids

These can be used, as with all the pad and shield drills, to build stamina but predominantly these exercises are used to build accuracy, technique and explosive speed. There are a number of ways of doing these and once you have the basics, you can work out your own variations.

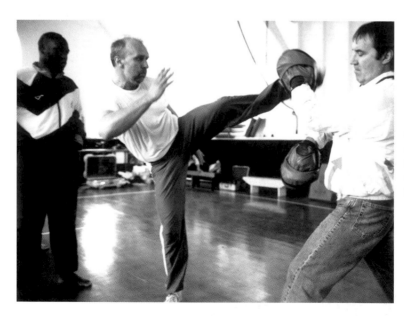

Your good self on left roundhouse, during the pyramid exercise, with others waiting for their turn.

First - decide how many techniques you are going to work up to at the top of the pyramid. Probably 5 is the maximum but 3 or 4 is okay. You need 3 - 4 people or more but restrict the number to 6. With one person holding the pads, the others line up facing him and behind each other. The range of techniques you are going to do have been pre-determined so everyone knows what he has to do.

The first time everyone goes through it is to perform on the first technique in the total of 5. For example, this could be a long, fast left jab. The last man through takes the mits or pads so as to allow the man who was initially holding them to take his turn.

The second time through, another technique is added, for example, left, high round-house kick. The third time through, the third technique, which could be a spinning back kick - right leg is added.
The fourth could have a right backfist added at the end of the spin and ---
The fifth technique could be a left low reverse punch to the stomach.
The pads are moved into position quickly for all 5 techniques to happen at speed.
The sixth time through, the technique, you drop the fifth technique, which was the low punch and only 4 are performed.
On the seventh, you are down to 3 and so on, until the last technique is the left leading jab you started with, done with explosion and aggression.
It's a taxing drill, but you have the ability to introduce spirit and aggression.

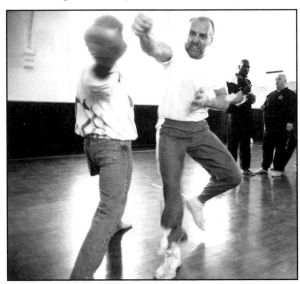

Finish your sequence on the pad pyramids with a big, aggressive shot and lots of noise.
In this case, it's a long distance 'blitz'.

Drill 8 - 50- Kick Rounds

One of the hardest kicking exercises. The target, as you've probably gathered, is to do 50 kicks, but how they are done is up to the 'pad man'. The pads can be hook & jab, Thai or the forearm pads. The pad man dictates the type and number of kicks. He can make it 5 kicks, 3 kicks or just one. The type of kicks are dictated by the positions the pads are held in. This still allows some freedom of choice by the kicker as he can vary the individual kicks to any particular signal.

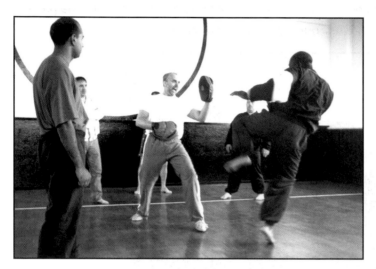

50-kick round. Everyone gathered round to give verbal support.

It is essential that the man with the pads keeps moving round, back and forward toward his partner so as to ensure good mobility at all times. From the kicker's point of view, he must not pace the kicks, but put everything, that is speed, accuracy, aggression and power into all his kicks.

Drill 9 - Pad - Chases

This drill is run as a 'shuttle' exercise, similar to wind sprints, only this time you are chased back to your start position by your partner. What is also included is that at each turn, there are a set number of kicks. The drill works something like this:

Both people are equipped with hook & jab mits, but don't worry if there are insufficient to go round, as you can use your hands for a focus point, providing there is correct control with the kicks. This does not have to be a 'power kicking' event, but is mainly speed, timing, accuracy and stamina building.

Both people face each other at approx. 15 metres, having predetermined the first series of kicks. This could be left front kick to the stomach, left high roundhouse kick, spinning back kick with the right leg and, possibly, a punch to finish. On the command, one person sprints to his partner and carries out the kicks - on completion he sprints back towards his starting position - this time followed by his partner. When he gets back to his start point, he turns quickly and puts the pads in position for his partner to carry out the kicking sequence.

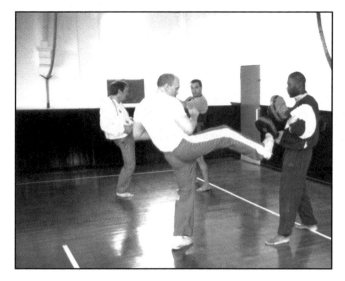

Pad Chases.

Above - the first man sprints to the pads and carries out the pre-arranged sequence.

Right - at the end of the sequence - both the attacker and his partner sprint back for the partner to carry out his sequence - and so on.

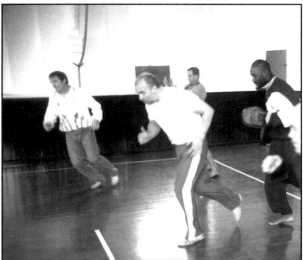

His partner turns, sprints back, followed by the first person and the sequence may be repeated so that each person has had 4-6 sprints and 4 kicking sessions - this is one set.

The kicking routine is changed and the sequence commenced again. For a complete drill, you would change the sequence some 4 times. Stay switched on, so that the moment you turn you have the pads quickly in position for your partner to commence his kicks. Don't 'amble' back after your kicks but turn and sprint quickly. The person who is chasing must encourage the person in front to push harder if he is lacking in sprint speed.

Drill 10 - Joint Bag Work

You can do the same thing as the pad pyramids, using a punch bag. This works on the same basis which is a line of people going through to do their techniques - the last man taking over the bag. This time, you have just 3 or 4 techniques to do on the bag and this could be just punches, kicks or both. One person holds the bag so it doesn't fly all over the place and makes the speed of combinations a possibility.

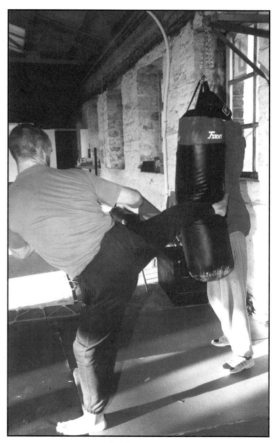

Joint bag work. When working fast, aggressive combinations on the bag, get your partner to hold it in position. He can also relay the degree of impact of the technique.

CHAPTER 10

PUTTING IT TOGETHER

By now, you may be more confused about what you should be doing - training wise - than ever before. Hopefully though, you'll have gained some new ideas, different approaches and some new drills to incorporate into your training.

For many, it's probably still and always will be a question of 'old dogs and new tricks', but approached with an open mind, everyone should find something of value. How should you combine the drills and exercises in this book? Unfortunately, there's no easy answer, because it solely depends on the imperatives you have that demand you are taken in one particular direction or other, with your training.

If you are still locked in, say, non-contact competition, you may need to 'lighten the load' with some of the more heavy and impactive drills in the book. You may also want to keep the work intense, but light and controlled. If your competition is of a more full contact nature, then you need to combine as many of the drills as you can. If you are reading this book, with little or no martial arts background, then many of the equipment drills will be confusing and overly difficult, but this should not prevent you from embarking on the whole range of 'stress drills' that I've illustrated.

Which Martial Art?

For those of you who are reading this book and who don't train in a martial art you are probably thinking that you need to rush out and get involved in some martial discipline so as to be able to kick pads and punch bags. Not a bad thought, but the enthusiasm needs tempering with some constructive thinking. No one martial art works for self defence. Those that are predominantly punching and kicking based are usually deficient in the grappling skills and vice versa. Most are highly complex and take years to get good at, but don't let competence stand in the way. Essentially pick any one and it will have a lot of what you are looking for. If you can, pick a club which is not 'Style' constrained. What I mean is find a club such as those we have in The British Combat Association which is more self defence and practically oriented.

Unfortunately on the fitness front, many martial arts systems are light. This is

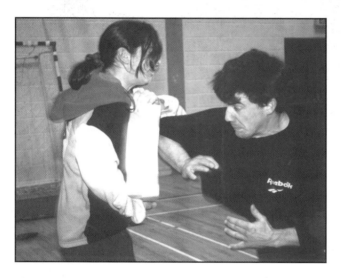

not the fault of the particular martial art, but the teacher who has come to realise that hard training does not go hand in hand with large classes. As he makes his money proportionate to the attendance - well the rest you can figure out for yourself.

A power - elbow strike onto an impact pad. This, for me, is where all training leads - Pre-Emptive Strikes. All training is a support system for this.

Combining the drills is a matter of balance. For example, there is no way I'm going to do more than 2 sessions of hill sprints training in one week. The demands it places on one's system are too great and it is unnecessary, particularly if you are also going to get a heavy 'leg' workout on the weights, at least twice in a 7-day period. What normally happens now in training books is that half of the book is made up of weekly training programmes, which vary everything and just fill space because they have little else to say. I'm not going to do that, but it's important that you try and combine types of training so as to vary the levels of intensity and endeavour to make them specific to your principle goal.

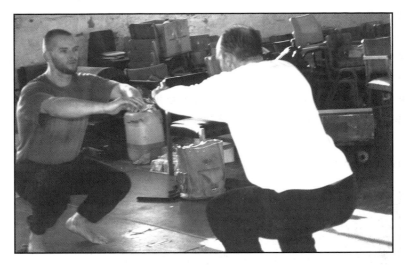

*Squats. 10 + 10. Tony Sykes impassively stares down yours truly - fortunate-
ly, my face and its pained expression is out of view.*
*The exercise is 10 slow squats, on the toes, with the arms held out in front, fol-
lowed by a slow count of 10 in the low position and so on for approx. 4 times.*

The emphasis will change, depending on your own motivation and the supply or not of training partners. Where you live, what equipment you have, will all dictate how you can mix and match the various cross-disciplines. Don't make excuses - no partners, no gym and no kit is no excuse - you can still run, sprint, punch and kick and work with and against your own body weight. Sissy squats, sit-ups and push-ups, plus chins, all work. Before now, I've hung small pieces of paper at various heights on strings from a washing line to create targets for punching. Surprisingly, they demand accuracy with a good snap and you can work fast, varied punches and combinations of punches, together with good body and head movements. It works and whatever the compromise, you are doing something.

One of the hardest sessions I've had in training was when Tony Sykes and I used to train on a football field. This of course, took place when there was no football match and we did this session probably twice in a week and often it could keep me awake the night before.

We started off - after a warm-up, with one of us setting off to sprint around the outside of the pitch. The other one then goes when his partner has completed a full circuit and touches him as he sprints past. The first to go gets a rest and as each circuit is just under a minute, this was the time of the rest period. This portion of the session would be repeated 3 - 4 times.

The second exercise was a full all-out sprint by one person from one end of the pitch to the other. When he crossed the far line at the end of the pitch, he put his arm in the air as the signal for his partner to go. His rest period again, was until his partner gets to him and then he sets off on a sprint back - the sequence again repeated for 4 sprints each. The final part is exactly the same exercise, but from the halfway line. The sprint should now be faster as its shorter, but so is the rest peiod - again repeat the dose for 4 times each.

At the end of this we were ready for the 'long sprint' - although ready is hardly the word I would have chosen at the time. This was a race against each other and was probably in the region of 400 metres +. After what we had done, with little rest, it is one of the most exacting sprints to do. The lactic acid, already present in the legs, soon builds up and you really felt you were running uphill, even on the flat.

Eventually, Tony and Bob Sykes transplanted the same exercise to an outdoor market in Huddersfield which was closed at night. It worked just as well and although shorter, it was faster as a circuit, with tighter turns and shorter rest periods. The long sprint was on a quiet stretch of road. The market was close to their dojo and was only part of an overall training session - hard it was!!

There's no such thing as a compromise really in training - just excuses. Make the most of what you've got - improvise and get stuck in. Even when you're driving around on other occasions, always keep a lookout for steps, hills, or potential circuits.

Don't expect to attract many like-minded people to such training regimes. It appeals to very few who are prepared to make that commitment to such hard and often distressing training routines. It will only ever be a small select few who'll pay their dues. But that's okay. If suddenly I found myself surrounded by hordes of willing training partners, I'd know that things had slipped and it had suddenly all got too easy. In the **'Fit to Fight' videos**, you can see some of the drills in action and the effort it takes. Whatever you do, and however you train, include one thing above all else - spirit.

In martial arts, its the one thing we have that stands out from all other sports or training disciplines - in

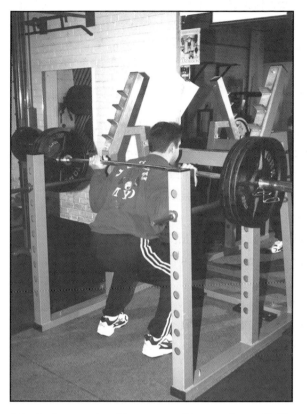

You don't get to be able to squat with reps of over 300lbs and strict, by making compromises in your training.

many ways 'spirit' is unique in the sense we use it in martial arts. Fighting spirit, training spirit, wherever it fits, it is very important it does fit. For many years, I've been aware that many of the more modern, freestyle, semi-contact fighters have technique and competitive flair, but in the training, lack spirit. This is not to say they have no fighting spirit, as they are highly combative, it is sometimes only a lack of spirit in the commitment to train and train hard.

I remember a quote from Sumo which was to the effect that **"we train until there is no sweat left"**, and it is that attitude, that spirit that needs to be inculcated into our training. In many ways, spirit is recognised as aggression. The two are the same, but in a way, aggression doesn't somehow serve to dignify the word and meaning of 'spirit'. Spirit is really epitomised by someone who is always ready to go, always ready to go first, always ready to take on more and always ready to encourage others in their efforts. Spirit is what separates simply 'doing' from 'feeling' and, I believe, sustains a trainer at times of low motivation.

Its also 'pride in performance' - never being satisfied with how you're training, but never showing negativity, especially if you're with others. If you are unhappy with your power or technique or combinations - keep it to yourself and sort it out.

"Train Hard - Fight Easy" - It's a trite and basically misleading statement. No fight is easy, even if it goes your way from the first split second. Fights are taxing mentally and physically and distressing. They hold within them all the consequences that physical confrontation involves, not least on occasions, the interest of the law. But all these must be pushed into a locked and inaccessible box - deep in one's unconsciousness at the time. Consequences must never be allowed to influence correct attitude and correct action in pre-emptiveness, when you are involved in a fight. Training can,

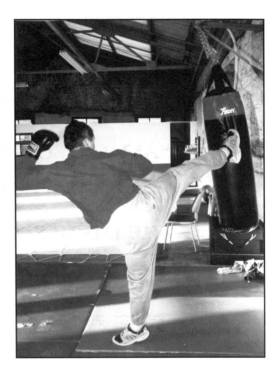

Spinning Back Kick. *Pinpoint accuracy from years of hard training and hard fighting.*

however, make a difference so much so that we can justifiably re-phrase the saying to read *'Train Hard - Fight Easier'* .

Success in any venture, of whatever nature, is usually based in direct ratio to our confidence to succeed and in this, we are victims of our sub-conscious programming - good or bad. This is where training and hard training comes in. By succeeding at hard training sessions, we are building the blocks of sub-conscious confidence. Surviving and achieving in a heavy session of sprints on the hill is a confidence-builder with few equals. If you can achieve a good performance, you know you are fit, strong, powerful, explosive and prepared and you also know you can last the distance should it ever go to one.

You know you are '**FIT TO FIGHT**'.

> # "ALL I GIVE YOU IS THE
> # OPPORTUNITY,
> # THE IMPULSE, THE KEY"
> ## (Herman Hesse)

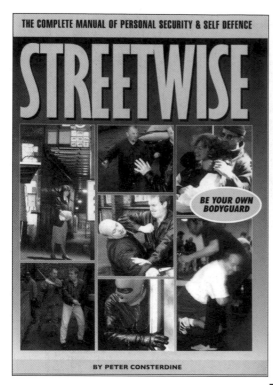

This manual is not another 'martial arts in jeans' type of self defence book. It combines detailed concepts from the world of bodyguarding, with the very best of self defence.

'Streetwise'
by
Peter Consterdine
£27.49
(inc. UK p & p)

The most complete book on the subject of Close Protection. 330 pages, over 100 photographs and numerous illustrations. Every subject explained in detail by one of the world's most experienced bodyguards.

'The Modern Bodyguard'
by
Peter Consterdine
£27.49
(inc. UK p & p)

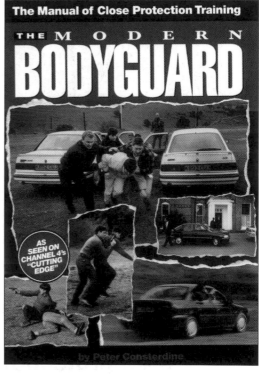

Peter is acknowledged as one of Britain's fittest martial artists.
A video not only for the martial artist, but for anyone who wants to be truly fit.

'Fit To Fight'
Video
by
Peter Consterdine
£26.49
(inc. UK p & p)

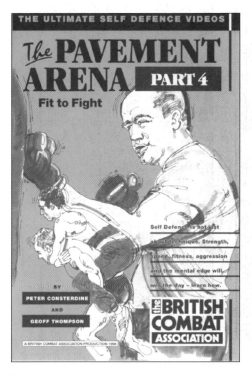

To order any of these products or for a **FREE** colour catalogue,
containing the full range of books and videos from
Protection Publications
please call our 24hr hotline

Telephone
0113 2429686
Major credit cards accepted

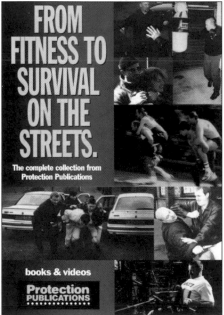

Visit our website on:-
www.protection-publications.co.uk